ENGINEERING THE ALPHA

ENGINEERING THE
ALPHA

A REAL WORLD GUIDE TO AN UNREAL LIFE

John Romaniello and Adam Bornstein

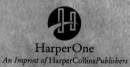

HarperOne
An Imprint of HarperCollinsPublishers

HarperOne

HarperCollins books may be purchased for educational, business, or sales promotional use. For information, please e-mail the Special Markets Department at SPsales@harpercollins.com.

HarperCollins website: http://www.harpercollins.com

HarperCollins®, ▇®, and HarperOne™ are trademarks of HarperCollins Publishers.

Designed by Terry McGrath
Illustration of "The Hero's Journey" on page 40 by Copter Labs.

FIRST HARPERCOLLINS PAPERBACK EDITION PUBLISHED IN 2014

Library of Congress Cataloging-in-Publication Data
Romaniello, John.
Engineering the alpha : a real world guide to an unreal life : build more muscle,
burn more fat, have more sex / by John Romaniello and Adam Bornstein. — First edition.
pages cm
ISBN 978-0-06-222089-9
1. Men—Health and hygiene. 2. Physical fitness. 3. Bodybuilding—Training.
I. Bornstein, Adam. II. Title.
RA777.8.R64 2013
613'.04234—dc23

2012047835

14 15 16 17 18 RRD(H) 10 9 8 7 6 5 4 3 2 1

For my mother, Linda Romaniello,
who taught me first to have strength,
and then how to use it,
and
Alvin Batista, my Obi-Wan,
who long ago gave me a book
sort of like this one.
—JR

To my parents—Ira and Sandy—who always understood
that being the Alpha was about becoming a better person and
helping others, and who raised me in a way that allowed
me to share that message with others.
—AB

Contents

Contents

Foreword

It started in the most primitive way you can imagine.

Before the championships or my move to America, and long before anyone talked about a Golden Age of bodybuilding, it began with a fantasy in the forests of Austria.

My friends and I imagined ourselves as gladiators. During the summer, we would charge up dirt trails all day, stopping to pound out sets of push-ups and squats. We would struggle through chin-ups on tree branches so thick our hands would slip off after the first few reps. And then, when we'd exerted ourselves, we would build a fire and cook our meat under the stars.

You could analyze the hell out of what led us to that particular fantasy. But if I had to guess, it was about escaping the depression that surrounded us by dreaming about men who created their own destiny by building their bodies, honing their skills, and, yes, engineering the Alpha.

The next summer, I would discover weights, and I was only a few years away from making my escape real by coming to America. The rest, you know.

That commitment to fitness that I developed as a young, imaginary gladiator has stayed with me all my life. After I won my titles, I wasn't content putting them on the shelf and walking away. I wanted to inspire others to join me in my fitness crusade.

When I began my career, if you asked someone where the nearest gym was, they would most likely look at you like you were a serial killer. If you were lucky, they would point you to some faraway dungeon with a few barbells and some weights.

Today, it's hard to find a strip mall or a building without a fitness center, and for the most part, you would never mistake a modern gym for a torture chamber. We've come a long way, but I know this is not a crusade that has an obvious end point. We will always have to keep pushing forward and fighting to show people the benefits of health.

I met Adam and Roman because they share my commitment to health and fitness. When I decided to get back into the fitness game, I sought out the best and brightest experts in the field. In that search, I asked everyone from my fans to my advisors who they recommended I look at. Without fail, the names Romaniello and Bornstein kept floating to the top. They've spent their careers inspiring people to live better lives. We got to know each other when they collaborated with me on my website to share the latest information and to spread our message as far as we can. For me, it's been an incredible experience. I've seen the fitness industry move from the workout pamphlets I used to staple together and walk to the post office to the lightning-fast sharing that happens over Twitter and Facebook. We can cast a much bigger net these days.

Within just a few months of connecting with Roman and Adam, I had applied some of their ideas to the oldest and most reliable testing ground I know: my own body. For me, it was very much like the old days, only instead of doing chin-ups on trees and hoping for results, I was using advanced concepts backed by science, methods to increase testosterone or manage insulin. I was using some of the concepts you will read about in this very book.

Adam and Roman are smart guys who are dedicated to expanding their knowledge so that they can help you improve. They know what they are talking about. I wouldn't have asked them to lead the charge with the fitness advice on my website if they didn't. If you follow what they've written in this book, you will be using advanced concepts backed by science; methods to increase testosterone or manage insulin.

This book, *Engineering the Alpha*, is the latest weapon in their arsenal. It is filled with information that can help you train more efficiently, melt fat as you build muscle, and harness your hormones to rediscover your inner Alpha. These two are the pioneers of the new wave of fitness. They are innovators who have worked tirelessly to discover new ways to motivate and continue the crusade that I started before they were born.

The research and methods contained here are cutting-edge, but the foundation is timeless. Every man, no matter how primitive, has dreamed of channeling his Alpha. It's a concept that goes beyond human evolution and explains the social hierarchies of the animal kingdom. But don't think this is about turning yourself into a silverback gorilla hybrid, pounding your chest as you ruthlessly intimidate your weaker counterparts.

It's about being happy, fit, and ready for anything. It's about finding your self-confidence and continuing to push yourself every day. It's about being hungry to be the best version of yourself.

Becoming the Alpha is different for every man. Maybe it's traveling across the Atlantic to become the world's best bodybuilder, becoming an actor or a politician, or even transforming into the gladiator you once dreamed of being. This is your shot at something bigger.

You picked up this book because you're searching for the same thing I was when I sat under the stars after a long day of big visions in the Austrian countryside. So turn the page and start finding it.

—*Arnold Schwarzenegger*

PART 1
INITIATION

"TAKE THE FIRST STEP, AND YOUR MIND WILL MOBILIZE ALL ITS FORCES TO YOUR AID. BUT THE FIRST ESSENTIAL IS THAT YOU BEGIN. ONCE THE BATTLE IS STARTLED, ALL THAT IS WITHIN AND WITHOUT YOU WILL COME TO YOUR ASSISTANCE."
—ROBERT COLLIER

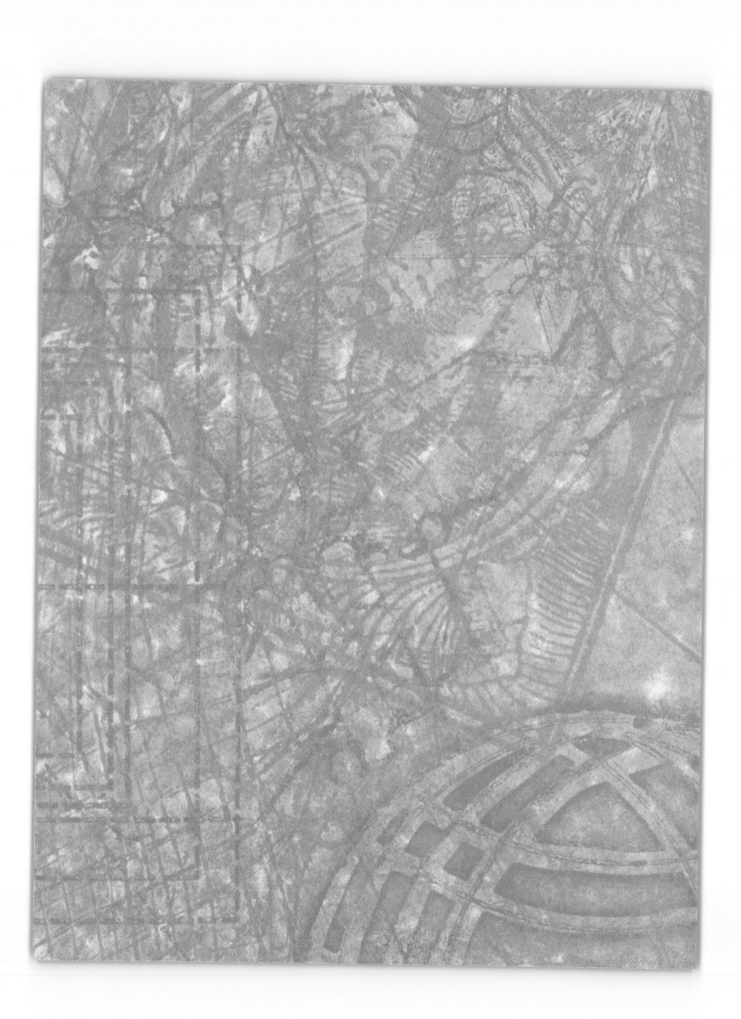

The Fall of Man

"The mass of men lead lives of quiet desperation."

—HENRY DAVID THOREAU

You are not your fucking khakis.*

You were built to be strong, fearless, confident, and powerful. You were designed to tame wilderness and carve canals through mountains, to conquer nations and build empires, to cross oceans and walk on the moon.

These are great things that great men can do and have done: achievements that require strength—and the wisdom to use it judiciously. While these examples loom large in history and may not seem immediately applicable to you, all men have what it takes to accomplish great things, and to be great themselves.

But examine the ordinary man and you wouldn't know it. Most men do not understand the levels of greatness they can achieve—not because they haven't tried—simply because they have no conception of the limitations they are facing, limitations they are creating.

The reason is a simple but hard-to-swallow truth: most guys unknowingly live their lives in an ordinary world with no thought to leave it.

---

* For those few poor souls who don't recognize it, this quote belongs to *Fight Club*'s Tyler Durden, a prototypical albeit hyperbolic Alpha who will be discussed later in this book.

Chances are, you are one of those guys.

This is not a judgment. We have no doubt that you bust your ass and strive for excellence. Of course you do; men, by nature, are driven to succeed and pursue greatness with their entire being. There's a certain swagger to being a man, a swagger that is built into your physiology and coded into your DNA—a swagger that is both created by ambition and simultaneously propels it.

But look at the ordinary man, and none of those traits are readily apparent. You don't see physical prowess; you see bad posture and high body fat. Talking to the ordinary man, you don't hear confidently spoken words giving voice to intelligent ideas; you hear clipped, half-developed thoughts, oftentimes expressed in a timid nature that undercuts the speaker's manhood.

The ordinary man is no longer impressive. We don't expect the ordinary guy to be particularly strong, particularly smart, or particularly fit—or successful, driven, funny, or confident. We don't *expect* him to be particularly anything.

These qualities are not expected of the ordinary, but they are the province of the Alpha. We expect these things of the Alpha—he's the one with the strength and the wit, the charm and the poise, the drive and the leadership.

Reading this, you might recognize in yourself a few of the qualities of the Alpha; perhaps you're already on the way to breaking away from ordinary, already engaged in a battle against typicality and mediocrity, working to become something more. It has no doubt occurred to some men reading this book that they can change, grow, and improve. Some. But not all. There are others who don't realize that they can change, or that they *should* change. They don't realize that they need to change. Some men are perfectly content in their universe.

Our warning isn't about happiness or comfort. We know—and hope—that many people reading this are living good lives. This book is about creating a fundamental recognition that as long as you live in the ordinary world, you are limited. And that by making some very small, strategic changes, you can trigger dramatic improvements to every aspect of how you live, the way you feel, your impact on others, and your health and wealth.

It's an undeniable reality that very few people are living the exact lives that they want, and that even fewer have advanced as far as they can physically, personally, and professionally. And we know that this book can help anyone get to the next level in any of those areas.

It's not about where you are in an absolute sense; it's about where you are relative to where you have the potential to be—and the sad truth is, very few men these days are living up to their potential.

It wasn't always this way.

THE RISE OF THE ORDINARY

So how did it all change? How did everything gravitate toward ordinary? How did the cultural avatar of manhood change from someone strong, confident, and ambitious to an unimpressive, milquetoast fellow with an obsequious* demeanor?

If you look at mankind over time—as we've moved from more capable to more dependent—the typical scapegoats aren't as much to blame as you probably think. Do increased food portions make us fat? Not according to a thirty-year study conducted by Harvard. (In reality, it's our snacking habits.) Is it a lack of time at the gym that has men carrying less muscle and suffering from more health problems like diabetes and heart disease? Hard to believe that's the issue when *more* men are spending time exercising than ever before. In fact, a Gallup Poll showed that nearly 50 percent of the population now exercises three or more times per week. And yet obesity rates are at an all-time high.

So why are so many men ordinary and so few Alpha?

There are several reasons that are typically not mentioned—ranging from sitting too much, to picking the wrong sexual partners, to not wearing the clothes that fit properly, to watching shitty reality TV. (Seriously.)

Think it's fucked up that clothes and reality TV are affecting men en masse? Just wait until you hear what it's doing to you personally. It really does start on an individual level.

Now, we understand that it might seem a little far-fetched that those things might affect your life so significantly. That anything so seemingly mundane as not standing often enough could have such a profound effect on your manhood. But please believe us—we have science to back this up.

Everything you do (or don't do) affects you both psychologically and physiologically. Every suit you wear, every book you read, every movie you watch is either edifying or eroding your ability to develop into the guy you want to be, the guy you know you can be—the guy who is the best version of you. Combine those with frequent bad food choices and inconsistent sleeping habits and we have all the elements of a dangerous recipe: a perfect storm of screw-ups leading to a universe where you are trapped—against your wishes or knowledge—in a cage of ordinary and a body that is not designed for excellence.

Taken collectively with your peers, those things—those seemingly innocuous choices—will be either the resurrection of true masculinity . . . or its complete demise.

Of course, we don't want that to happen. In fact, we've already seen enough great men held back by limitations they didn't even know existed. Those are real problems, and we'll cover each and every one of those things in stark detail in this book. Our goal is to make sure that those issues no longer exist in your life. And that your only concerns are wonder-

---

* Yeah, we just used *milquetoast* and *obsequious* in the same sentence. In addition to changing your life, this book will make you awesome at Scrabble.

ing why you didn't make these changes sooner and why you ever believed some of the lies in the fitness industry that we'll share in this book. Those are Alpha problems—regrets from your past that indicate a better present and a greater future. And when you become the Alpha, that's the type of universe you create: one of contentment, a lack of frustration, and a confidence that you control who you are, what you look like, and what you can achieve.

BECOMING THE ALPHA

Listen, we fully realize that some of this might sound like doom and gloom or a condescending appraisal of your life. Let's kill that thought right now. This book is not a judgment of who you are, what you have accomplished, or your level of happiness. This is a reality check on a global level.

We've been fully invested in the health and wellness industry for more than a decade, and we've seen a disturbing trend that has yet to be addressed. We're not here to point the finger at the same issues, such as carbs, fat, lack of activity, and misleading fad diets. Following that same old song and dance is like trying to track down Keyser Söze.* The solution has been under our nose the entire time. The reason nothing has changed is that we've pursued the wrong enemy.

The real culprits are behavioral decisions and lifestyle choices that have disrupted the functioning of your hormones. This is the stealth bomber of the health industry because guys aren't made aware they can *naturally* control their hormones. More importantly, no one seems to stress how much your hormones control how you look, feel, and age. Today's diets and exercise programs have played their role in creating a society full of men suffering from hormonal dysfunction.

Without knowing it, you're suffering from lower testosterone, dwindling levels of growth hormone (GH), and high amounts of stress-induced cortisol.

Yeah . . . *you.*

As in, every single man who hasn't made a conscious effort to improve hormonal functioning. (Oh, and did we mention you might *also* be pumping out estrogen like a pregnant woman?)

It's the pink elephant in the room that no one seems to acknowledge: doctors, trainers, nutritionists, and mainstream media ignore the fact that society has developed in a way that's led to a downshift in our hormones, making us less manly.

In fact, the only place you'll see any acknowledgment of this phenomenon is in the pharmaceutical industry—and that's because they just want to sell you a drug to fix it. While that would just be treating the symptom (and ultimately be counterproductive), at

---

* If you haven't seen *The Usual Suspects* recently, do yourself favor and watch the film. Kevin Spacey tries to go all Alpha in *American Beauty*, but this is probably his best role.

least Big Pharma recognizes what nearly everyone else seems to miss: hormones are really the key to everything.

Hormones are what make you a man. What enable you to be the Alpha. And their suboptimal functioning is the reason why men have evolved into the ordinary.

It's not only logical but also undeniable that hormonal dysfunction is the reason men are fat, slow, weak, indecisive, or overly emotional. Maybe all of the above. It's the reason men are uninterested—or, perhaps worse, uninteresting—when it comes to sex. More than that, it's endangering overall health, messing with your confidence, and compromising libido in terms of both enjoyment and conception.

In short: hormonal dysfunction is the silent killer of the fundamental attributes that make you a man. It's what's undermining your potential to be the Alpha.

If men knew the true impact of hormonal optimization and that they could influence their hormones naturally, then every guy would spend more time trying to fix the very essence of what makes him a man, right?

That's exactly what you'll discover in this book. You're going to learn about all of the individual hormones you can impact, including testosterone, GH, estrogen, leptin, ghrelin, and cortisol. You're going to learn the potential risks of hormonal imbalances as well how to identify them. Perhaps most importantly, you'll learn how to correct them.

We're going to show you how to recognize and fix these issues, all while losing fat, building muscle, and increasing your sex drive. We're going to teach you these things by adjusting the way you eat and the way you train—but we're also going to help you understand how all these things go far beyond the physical world.

We're going to prove—with science and real world results—how getting stronger in the gym can help strengthen your character and how strategically pigging out while watching football can make you better in bed. (No, we're not fucking with you.)

This book will give you an understanding about how to become a better you—a better person—inside and out.

This isn't just a fitness book. It's a road map that brings together all the elements that are important to you. This book will give you an understanding about how to become a better you—a better person—inside and out. We're approaching this through fitness because we've discovered that for most men, the first step toward mastery of the self should be mastery of the body. And hormones hold the key.

So yes, we *are* going to cover getting bigger biceps and *hawt abz*. And you're absolutely going to get a number of amazing workouts, pick up new exercises, and learn the most cutting-edge dietary strategies in the world. But we're going to cover these subjects in a way that will cut through the typical bullshit that bombards your life, stalls your progress, and limits your results. We're going to cover everything in a way that unites the science with the practical application—a way that ties physicality with social, emotional, and

ENGINEERING THE ALPHA

SUBJECT: *Claudio Espinoza*

THE ORDINARY WORLD

I have always been trapped in the body of a chubby kid, and as such, I suffered the usual embarrassments of not taking my shirt off at the beach in the summer, wearing ill-fitting clothes, and a bruised ego that would make it difficult to approach the opposite sex. At times, I would grow tired of feeling this way and I would hit the weight room, but my interest in working out rarely translated to permanent lifestyle changes.

ACCEPTING THE CALL

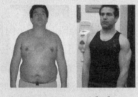

After turning thirty I said, "No more!" Having gone from a chubby kid to a borderline-obese adult, I knew I'd have my work cut out for me. I found Roman, a kindred spirit who understood what it was like to look in the mirror and know, "I'm better than this!"

Roman provided me with all the tools and encouragement necessary to transform, both inside and out. Following his recommendations allowed me to lose almost twenty pounds of fat within the first six weeks. That was my initial goal and we still had five months left!

ALPHA STATUS

Every week I could see the fat being whittled away, and in its place was solid muscle. My strength on all lifts doubled, if not tripled. By the end of our program, I was able to see my abs! I went from 217 pounds to 173 pounds, losing about 50 pounds of fat and gaining about 10 pounds of muscle. While there was more to be done, I knew that Roman would be there for me, continuing to mentor and guide me along as I continued to hone in on my desired physique.

In doing this, I inspired several friends to take positive steps to take charge of their lives and bodies. I can say in no uncertain terms that this has been the most rewarding aspect of my physique transformation. Thanks to me, many friends began to wonder if they too could follow in my footsteps and take control of their body, with some even embarking on their own transformations. Now I feel like I have many of the necessary tools to continue building the body I've always wanted and help others to achieve their physique transformation goals.

cognitive development, all brought together under a single umbrella of hormonal balance* and life enhancement.

We're not trying to sell what's in our book. We're firing a warning shot from a cannon. And at this point, you have two choices.

You can forget everything you just read. You can ignore the *obviousness of the truth*.** You can pretend that you don't understand that your body and your mind, your ambition and your sex drive, your waist and your wallet are all being assaulted by hormonal dysfunction. You can disregard our promise of providing you with a new plan specifically intended to do one thing: lead you step-by-step to becoming the best possible version of yourself. And you can set this book down and walk away from the road map created for the sole purpose of engineering the Alpha.

Or you can keep reading with a complete understanding that what you hold in your hands isn't just a manual for getting into the greatest shape of your life—it's a real world guide to an unreal life.

Choose wisely.

---

*If you *don't* want the science . . . well, that's weird to us. But we're geeks. Maybe you just want the results. That's fine. Skip to part 3 for the workout and diet plans. Whether you read this entire book from the intro to the afterword or just skip to the parts about sex and training, the result will be a better body, mind, and sex life.

**This phrase was pirated directly from *The Matrix*, in a scene that fittingly mirrors this one: Morpheus is attempting to explain the Matrix to Neo. At that point, Neo does not yet realize either the seriousness of the situation or his potential. For some readers, this could not be more fitting.

THE BOOK NO ONE HAS WRITTEN

"If you're gonna write a book . . . write a fuckin' book."

—*TIM FERRISS*

■ *ENTER ROMAN*

If you really want to hear about it,* *when I decided to write a book, I figured it should be the one I always wanted to read. Ideally, the one that would have changed things for me. It would be the book that—if only I'd been able to get my hands on it—would have saved me a lot of time, a lot of money, and probably a lot of headaches. Which is what I'd like to do for you.*

This book would have helped me achieve success a lot faster. It would have helped me get a better body in less time. It would have taught me that while there's no right way to train, there are a lot of wrong ways and I could go farther faster by avoiding them. This book would have helped me understand nutrition, understand food in a way that allows for freedom and ease. It would have taught me to be more confident and how to use that confidence to improve my friendships, avoid screwing up with women, and even achieve a higher sense of purpose.

But I didn't have it. Instead, I had to do things the hard way, learn things the hard way. I had to do the research and test the methods. I had to make mistakes. Over the past twelve years, I've made a ton of them—but also had a lot of successes.

As a coach, I've helped many people make their bodies look and perform better than they thought possible—everyone from athletes to actors and actresses to the nine-to-five businessman and the housewife. As a writer, I've published hundreds of articles in dozens of publications, served on the advisory boards of some of the largest fitness companies in the world, and now written this book.

The successes were fun, but the failures were probably more valuable. Because it's through those failures and the lessons learned that I was forced to stray from conventional methods and to develop the information in this very book.

---

* *Out of interest, these are the opening words of, and a direct homage to,* The Catcher in the Rye, *a book for which Roman has an unrepentant affection.*

■ *CHANGING YOUR PERCEPTION*

The largest mistake I made was not a single event or decision but rather a misguided view of the world that led me through most of the early part of my life: a worldview made up of a strange mix of insecurity and narcissism. I was caught in a mind-set and a perspective through which I drew value only through external factors. This limited me in a number of profound ways, the most damaging of which was my assessment of self: my self-worth was based on other people—on what they thought and on measuring myself against them.

When it came to anything, whether it was school, sports, or eventually work, I wasn't concerned so much with how I was doing as I was with where I fell in a hierarchy—how I was doing compared to others.

Of course, I didn't really know I was doing this. I just knew that no matter how well I did, I never really felt satisfied. It wasn't until I approached my late twenties, standing on a stage in my underwear, that I had an epiphany.

Here's how it happened: For a few years, I competed in bodybuilding, and although I won one of my shows and placed in the others, I found the competitions unsatisfying. I couldn't figure out why—until my last contest. I was standing on stage with three other guys, all tanned and oiled up, flexing and posing and doing their best Arnold impressions. And suddenly, for no reason I can name, a switch flipped and it stopped being fun.

Bodybuilding itself was enjoyable, but bodybuilding competitions did nothing for me. I began to realize that the idea of the competitions was what bothered me. It was the need to quantify and create competition in something that is very much an individualist endeavor. The dieting and extreme attention to detail appealed to me. Getting bigger than I had previously been was enticing and motivating. So was getting leaner. But comparing myself to other big or lean people wasn't a draw. This was the first in a series of realizations that begat a paradigm shift and allowed me to see things differently.

Up until that point, like many guys, I had been solely consumed with progress as it applied to advancement—within a sports team, a business setting, or even a social environment. I realized that I had fallen prey to the idea of beating everyone else.

Wanting to be better than other people is a fundamentally bankrupt concept; you'll quickly realize that you can't be better than everyone in the world, not at everything—and if being better than others is the source from which you draw happiness, there is no scenario in which you'll be truly happy. While that seems obvious to me now, it's an idea that escaped me for much of my life. And I think it escapes many men worldwide.

I was far too consumed with buying into the concept of what it meant to be the alpha male, when I should have been focused on becoming the Alpha me.

Before we move any farther, it's important that you understand what we're offering by transforming you into the Alpha. Like any partnership—and this is a partnership—there should be complete transparency for what's at stake.

We understand that the word Alpha *carries with it certain connotations. And in order for you to fully grasp our meaning and definition, we must first strip away any preconceived thoughts that are tied to that term.*

The general perception of an alpha male is someone who's, well, kind of an asshole. The guy who's strong and confident but also domineering and cocky. As it is currently understood, the alpha male tears down others as a means to elevate his own status. We stereotype this archetype as the good-looking quarterback who picks on nerds. It's the domineering middle management boss who publicly castigates his employees to assert his power. Of course, the stereotypical perception is not always the reality. A lot of quarterbacks are really nice guys. So are a lot of bosses.

The alpha male—in current context—is a troubling mix of generally positive traits that are executed in a negative way. We see this manifest itself in many instances of life. The biggest and strongest kid in school chooses to become the bully rather than someone who sets the best example. The men from small beginnings work the hardest and rise to the top—only to forget their humble beginnings.

Being good *doesn't mean you* are *good. So the goal is not about identifying good (being hardworking) or desirable (being strong) traits, but it is about understanding how to draw the line between Alpha and ignorant.*

Part of the reason for the negative perception of being the Alpha is how prevalent that word is in the seduction or pickup-artist community. Within that world, the drive to be the Alpha comes from an understanding that adopting certain traits might enhance your ability to get laid. While there's nothing wrong with getting laid or putting yourself in a better position to do so, that's not the point we're trying to make.

The entire foundation of pickup-artist society draws its self-worth by comparing to other people. More to the point, the idea of being Alpha in that community is not at all based on personal improvement; it's based on comparative improvement. It's a hollow approach to motivation.

We want to take back the concept of the Alpha. Consider this a rebranding campaign designed to get back to the roots of the meaning. Guys should desire to be the Alpha. Accepting this new perception will help you more clearly define the positive traits you want to possess and guide you toward the type of man you want to be.

For us, the issue with the perception of the alpha male is not that he's boorish* and kind of a bully; the issue is that it's a label that draws its power from others. And that's not how you create success.

So who is the Alpha? The Alpha is someone who is not just assertive but is also evolved.

We believe that the Alpha is the most evolved version of you. This is not about being the AMOG—the Alpha Male of the Group. That's an unfulfilling approach. Just think about it. Your mind-set isn't "I want to be good" or "I want to be better." It's "I want to be better than the other guys in the room." That approach makes it hard to ever feel satisfied or experience the positive feelings that come with achievement and success. Your goals should be based on your own expectations, not on something as abstract and unpredictable as who else is in the room.

We want you to focus on what you can control.

Competition is great. But the best indicator of success is always internal motivation. Think about the most successful people in the world. Their hustle and determination is never about living up to someone else's expectations or following in the footsteps of another. It's about blazing their own path, being unique, and becoming the first of their kind. Kareem was Kareem. Magic was Magic. Jordan was Jordan. And LeBron is LeBron. The comparisons will be inevitable, but none of these individuals preset their development based on someone else's plan.

We want you to judge yourself against only yourself. We want you to achieve success that you strive for, that you want, constantly trying to improve internally and externally because you want to be better than you were—not better than someone else. That is being the Alpha.

If you can't understand that your goals shouldn't be dependent on how you compare to others, then you will have difficulty reaching the goals you desire and living a fulfilled life.

---

* Yeah, boorish; like we said, you're going to get really good at Scrabble.

"The young man knows the rules, but the old man knows the exceptions."
—OLIVER WENDELL HOLMES

The funny thing about getting older is you learn that some of the things you used to hate are what you really need the most. Take rules for example. No guys actually like rules. We spend most of our lives bending them, breaking them, and genuinely disrespecting them in every way possible . . . that is, until we realize our brazen behaviors have left us without a fundamental mentality that guides who we are and what we can become.

Many guys feel that rules are restrictive. In reality, the right rules give you freedom. They allow you to make time for what you really need to do to become an Alpha. That's why we created the Alpha Rules. They sit just far enough outside of society's rules that you can live the life you want, and yet they still provide guiding principles that anyone can respect.

But this list is only the beginning. We encourage you to create your own set of rules. Part of being an Alpha is setting your own standards and principles and sticking to them. So we encourage you to write down your rules and add to the list. But here's the law: you must follow those rules. If you choose to set a standard by which you want to live, then you must actually follow through. Doing so will help ensure that your life doesn't lead down a path to the ordinary.

Rule #1. Make time for what's important. *Everyone* is busy, but there's a huge difference between being busy and being productive. Alphas are willing to sacrifice small things for important ones, even if it means giving up a little fun.

Rule #2. Consider the problem from all angles to find a solution. Alphas know that sometimes you need a hammer, other times a key. Developing an understanding of how to address problems is an infinitely valuable life skill.

Rule #3. Embrace ego as a mechanism to become more confident. But ego should never prevent you from listening to others or being willing to learn. Alphas are always open to the idea that they can learn more.

Rule #4. Understand the importance of sex. Alphas want sex to be meaningful to them in a number of ways. Whether you quantify that by performance or connecting with your partner, great sex is something that Alphas are great at. Put somewhat less delicately, Alphas are fucking *great* at fucking.

Rule #5. Say no to things you don't like.

Rule #6. Don't ask permission—beg for forgiveness (it's easier).

Rule #7. Don't criticize an idea unless you're willing to provide an alternative.

Rule #8. Get your clothes tailored. A $200 suit that fits well looks better than a $500 suit that doesn't.

Rule #9. Show love. Never, ever, ever hold back from giving a compliment, as long as it's sincere. There's never a bad time to say something nice; get in the habit of doing this. People will love you for it.

Rule #10. Always be the first to reach for the check. Do this even if the other person invited you out. If he or she puts up a strong fight, let 'em have it. Alphas try to take care of others and never want to be beholden to anyone, but they don't force dominance on other people, especially financially.

Rule #11. Answer all insults with a smile. Alphas understand that not everyone is going to like them, and some people will be vocal about it. There's no point giving them the satisfaction of giving a shit.

Rule #12. Admit your mistakes with honesty and humor. Accepting responsibility for your actions, especially when they're mistakes, is vitally important. Alphas do this, and they always go the extra step to make things right.

Rule #13. Take the lead. Always suggest a day and time to meet instead of leaving it in the air. Alphas don't wait for others to suggest things—they make things happen.

Rule #14. Understand that scared money don't make money. This is an old saying that is common in the poker world, and it's another way of saying "fortune favors the bold." Alphas take risks and savor both the sweetness of victories and the lessons learned in defeat.

Rule #15. Learn how to cook. If you're approaching thirty and you can't make a few meals, take the next month and learn. Seriously, time to grow the fuck up. Alphas know how to feed themselves. It's a basic human function.

CHAPTER 1

The Fitness Industry Is Completely Fucked Up

ENTER ADAM: UNMASKING THE FAÇADE OF EVERYTHING PUBLISHED IN THE MAINSTREAM

"You want answers? You can't handle the truth!"

—*A FEW GOOD MEN*

You want to know what the problem is with being an editor for the most-read fitness publications in the world, as I am?

You might think it's the low pay, the ninety-hour workweeks, and the complete anonymity that comes with not having your name on 95 percent of the stuff you write. All reasonable guesses, but that stuff isn't so bad when you get to work with some of the smartest people in the world, learn the best ways to improve your life, and train with athletes who are even cooler and more badass than they appear on TV.

The real problem: it's really hard to do my job the way it should be done. It's bullshit, and I'm tired of it. And I've finally reached a point where I'm ready to call out the industry because it's time for a fucking change.

Is this a rant? No. It's a much-needed stand that will explain why most guys never see the type of results promised and why you are actually capable of achieving much more than you probably think.

The fitness industry is just like the food industry—or any industry, for that matter. The truth is always hiding somewhere between what you see and what you believe.

How do I know? I've been part of the process that created the problem, and I have been diligently working to find a solution. And what I discovered was that in order to fix a broken system, we needed to introduce a little chaos.

That chaos is *hormones*.

Not the steroids and antiaging clinics that make everyone think of José Canseco and doping controversies. There's nothing controversial about what we'll share—but the end game is just as salacious and headline grabbing. And if we should remember Canseco for anything, it's that he shed light on a reality that was overlooked by all: people who focus on hormones age better, look better, and perform the way they want.

But you don't need a chemistry set to become superhuman. You can achieve that *naturally*. No pills, no shots, no injections. As we've already mentioned, the benefits go far beyond looking fucking awesome. Your hormones are the key to optimizing physical, social, and cognitive performance. This is basic endocrinology that's sixty years of research in the making—only no one has the balls to talk about it.

Until now.

No one's talking about it because the fitness industry is not an open forum for discussion. It's close-minded, dogmatic, and really confusing. It's no wonder most guys are unsure about what they should eat, when they should eat, and the best way to exercise. And if your health weren't the crux of everything in life, this wouldn't be a big deal.

But your health directly influences everything in your life. And we mean *everything*—your wealth, happiness, intelligence, sex life, and longevity. And that's just the short list. Every aspect of how you live and feel depends on the way you exercise and what you eat. But you don't hear that from the media. You just see the same cover lines: "Build Bigger Biceps," "Get Back in Shape," and "Six-Pack Secrets."

But I have a question: How are those headlines working out for you?

BEHIND THE FEAR

The information you receive from the mainstream media is somewhat designed to help you achieve those goals of bigger biceps and firmer six-packs. But they all miss the bigger picture. Larger biceps aren't about doing curls. Getting back in shape isn't about getting the cardio in. And having a six-pack isn't about not eating after seven P.M. That's a bullshit sundae topped with enough restrictions to drive anyone to the late-night Dairy Queen in a way that blows up your best-laid plans.

I'm sorry, but you've been screwed.

You don't get the results the media offers—but you do get plenty of frustration. This is because the gatekeepers in the fitness world would rather be consistent than progressive. They assume they know what the readers want, and therefore the information you receive is always pushed through a selective filter.

This leaves us with a frustrating reality: information spread by the mainstream media that is oftentimes designed to maintain the status quo rather than be completely transparent.

That's because people don't like admitting they're wrong—or just not completely right. Oftentimes what prevents personal growth is narrow-mindedness, not outright stubbornness. For whatever reason, they're unwilling to make changes to their value system.

What does it all mean? You've been fucked over with half-truths. I won't call them lies, but they *are* deceptions. Most of what is assumed to be the foundation of fitness just isn't all that accurate. That's not to say that none of it works—but not all of it is likely to be information that will work for you. And that's why you're stuck with the same frustrating thoughts about your body, your life, and your confidence.

This is partly human nature and partly culture: whether you want to admit it or not, changing your mind is seen as weakness, even though we know that sometimes the best decisions require us to let go of a previously held belief and accept a new mind-set that is better. But our refusal to change easily occurs because of the backlash that is associated with shifting your stance.

When politicians shift positions, they're called flip-floppers; when musicians do it, they're called sellouts. In the fitness industry, it's a little different. There's no gentle term, so they're just called idiots. They are decried for their inconsistency and accused of changing their message to suit a hidden agenda or to sell a product.

Despite the idea that this industry is supposedly propelled by science and research—which should be absorbed and applied to an ever-changing understanding of the human body—the truth is that it's not. Unfortunately, people would rather be comfortable with familiar ideas that they believe to be true than be challenged with new ideas that actually force them to think. The comfort in these beliefs creates a dogmatic view that paralyzes your ability to move forward.

As men, we hit a wall because the information we received, the advice we accepted, and the fitness and diet programs we welcomed into our life limited what we could achieve and who we could become.

We're tired of it all. You deserve more.

That's why I've spent several years working to create a blueprint—combining science with real life results—to prove how the truth was really being kept from you.

Is this a fuck-you to the fitness industry? Nah. But it *is* a stand that's long overdue. This is the first time anyone in the mainstream is taking a more open and honest approach, tackling the topics no one discusses, debunking the myths that are ruining your body, and opening your eyes to a world where sensational cover lines can be actual goals, not a marketing sell.

We are here to change the game, but not with the same old rigmarole; the only thing I can guarantee about this new world is that it won't be one filled with half-truths and empty promises.

LOOK (AND FEEL . . . AND FUCK) LIKE A REAL MAN

While we understand that much of the excitement you have for this book is probably tied to the workouts and diet plans, it's important to understand why we've written this book and exactly what's at stake. A bad hormonal environment is a Molotov cocktail waging war on your body. When your body isn't functioning optimally, you only experience the symptoms. Rarely do you understand the cause. That's why we will connect the dots so you understand how your daily behaviors set off an easily prevented domino effect of problems you desperately want to avoid.

We've listed nine problems that can be easily avoided if you fix your hormones. Some might be impacting you now, whether you know it or not. Others inevitably wait in the future. And all of them can be removed from your reality. If you didn't need your eyes to read, we'd tell you to close them now. Because this shit is about to get scary.

1. Reduced Intelligence

You might think most of the benefits of hormone optimization relate to how you look and feel. And you'd be right—fix your hormones and you will look awesome. But hormonal imbalance also impacts your brain. More specifically: not targeting your hormones through diet and training means less intelligence and a limited capacity for achievement.

The key is a hormone called BDNF—one of the biggest scientific advances that no one is talking about. What it stands for (brain-derived neurotrophic factor) isn't as important as what it means because if you don't produce more BDNF, it could stand for "brain does not function."

The concept is best understood this way: Have you ever seen the movie *Limitless* with Bradley Cooper? In it, Cooper's character takes a pill that maximizes brain functioning. He becomes brilliant—not because he suddenly has more knowledge but because his brain is firing and operating at a more efficient pace. This is BDNF.

When you're not cranking out enough BDNF, your brain is functioning on an average level like everyone else's, and your ability to become smarter is limited by the number of synapses you create. Fewer synapses mean less brain activity. But when BDNF is activated? It's like "Miracle-Gro for the brain," says Dr. John Ratey, associate professor of clinical psychiatry at Harvard Medical School. Become better looking *and* smarter? It's true, but we're just starting to scratch the surface.

2. Stunted Sex Drive

Having sex once a week isn't normal.

Here's the sad truth: there's a nation of guys out there with beautiful girlfriends (or boyfriends) or wives. Girlfriends and wives who want sex every night. This isn't the sad part, obviously. The sad part is that these guys, who should be counting their blessings—and having more sex than is advisable or safe—are falling asleep in front of the TV. Or lying in bed, staring at the ceiling, waiting for their partner to doze off.

These men love their girlfriends, love their wives, and on some level love sex. They just don't want it. Their sex drive, once a proud engine that influenced every decision, now has the power of a toy car with a dying battery.

Declining sex drive is a direct effect of lower testosterone, and it's not normal. It's not okay. It should be a very obvious indicator that you need to make a change. Put in the most blunt terms possible: You're a *man*, man.* If you don't want to fuck, something is wrong.

Some might write this off as one of the natural signs of aging. And to some extent, that's true. However, falling testosterone is no longer solely the province of middle age alone. Whereas you might expect a guy in his fifties to experience what the pharmaceutical companies call "Low T." This is happening to guys as young as twenty-five. Yes—there are a host of guys just out of college who don't want sex.

Even worse, new research from Australia has found that declining testosterone is not as much a result of aging as we once thought. Your decline in hormonal production is actually the result of your health and your body fat. "It is critical that doctors understand that declining testosterone levels are not a natural part of aging and that they are most likely due to health-related behaviors or health status itself," says Gary Wittert, MD and study coauthor.

The good news: this is easy to fix for guys young and old. While we can't promise that you'll have the same sex drive at forty-eight as you did at eighteen, it is possible to naturally increase your levels of testosterone—and thereby your sex drive—without pills or creams or doctors. We can tweak them with the right training approach. It's not lifting weights—it's how you lift them and when you lift them. Mix that with some nutrition secrets that you won't find on the cover of your favorite magazine, and you have a potent cocktail that primes you for less fat and more confidence, resulting in more testosterone and, even better, more incredible sex.

3. Accelerated Aging

Listen, we're not going to call you old and slow. But odds are, your body looks a lot older and moves a lot slower than it should. And it doesn't matter if you're a twenty-year-old guy or a sixty-year-old boss; the nutrition advice you've received is creating an impending apocalypse within your body.

You've probably heard of cleanse diets—most likely from your wife or girlfriend, or if you were trying to pass a drug test. (Yeah, we know why you really visit your favorite

---

* Other ways to make this point would have included, "You're a *bro*, bro," and "You're a *dude*, dude." Please select the one that sits best with your vernacular and self-identification.

supplement store.) These are the juice cleanses or liver and kidney detoxifiers that are supposed to rid your body of toxins, improve the functioning of your internal organs, and help you age better. Or, at the very least, you'll eat more fruits and vegetables and be a little healthier. But mostly it's just a marketing scheme to get you to buy a product.

The only *real* cleanse occurs at the cellular level. It's called autophagy, and it's your body's ability to regenerate and become better. Autophagy helps you repair injuries, makes your brain function a little better, helps with muscle growth and fat loss, and even assists in your ability to walk and breathe.

You see, every day there are millions of cellular reactions occurring in your body. Some of this activity causes damage within your body. As with any equipment that is used a lot, the daily stress causes breakdown. Fortunately, your body is built for such circumstances and can naturally heal anything that isn't working at an optimal level. This is autophagy.

So what happens when your internal repair is slow and lazy and doesn't get the job done? That's when you have a damaged internal environment. More specifically, when your workers don't repair your mitochondria—the cellular power plant of your body—then your body is basically fucked.

You age faster. You suffer from chronic disease. You lose your hair. And you get fat.

That brings us back to hormones. Your lack of growth hormone (GH) is limiting the natural process of autophagy. And as your GH levels continue to sputter along, your tissue continues to degenerate. It's why you have more aches and pains. Why food seems to make you fatter than it used to. And why muscle just won't appear on your body, no matter how many reps and sets you perform.

What's the best way to pump up your GH and turn the autophagic process into a group of grind-it-out interns that will work when needed? Strategic eating.

This isn't about specific foods or how many grams of protein, carbs, and fats you eat. It's simpler than that. This is about when you eat. Or more specifically, when you don't eat. The more time you spend eating—as in actual hours during the day eating—the less time you spend in the autophagic process.

That's why we'll teach you when you should and shouldn't be eating. It offers you the freedom to still eat the foods you love and follow the diet of your choice—whether it's low-carb, vegan, or meat-eater's delight (our personal favorite).

By turning on autophagy at the right time, you'll be stripping off fat in ways you didn't think possible and speeding the muscle-gain process. Just as importantly, your brain will work more efficiently, and research shows that you can even fight off diseases such as Parkinson's and Alzheimer's. Autophagy will change your life, your mind, and your body in ways that will have your internal organs working like a machine and your reflection looking like a man.

4. Lack of Sleep

We don't want to bore you, but you need more sleep. Why? It's simple: lack of sleep is associated with:

★ **More fat**

★ **More hunger**

★ **Smaller muscles**

★ **More irritability**

★ **Higher stress**

★ **Earlier death**

Not sure about you, but none of that sounds good to us, especially the death part.

We've made some calls and tried to get more hours added to the day—but that hasn't worked. So we realize that you might not always be able to achieve seven or eight hours of sleep per night. You're busy. We get it. But that's not a good enough excuse.

Take a hard look at the end-of-evening activities you can cut out to get to bed an hour earlier. Do you really need to check Facebook again? Is it imperative to catch up on ESPN *right now*? Cut things off a bit early and head to bed.

If you're still not convinced, here's what's more important to understand about your nightly ritual: it's not necessarily how long you sleep, but the quality of your sleep that is directly correlated to improving your life and health on a daily basis, say researchers at the Institute of Medicine. While there are numerous studies that show a link between poor sleep and diseases such as hypertension and diabetes—as well as shorter life span—this study focused on the problems that sleep causes in your day-to-day life. And after reviewing the behaviors and self-reported tendencies of more than ten thousand people, a connection is very clear: lack of sleep ruins your ability to function. You have trouble concentrating, remembering information, driving, taking care of your finances, and performing your job at a high level. And those were just the top five problems associated with a lack of sleep.

While none of this may sound shocking, what's most interesting is how easily you can change how you feel. The survey found that more than 30 percent of adults sleep less than six hours per night. And these people were the ones with the highest percentage of related problems. Those who slept more than eight hours per night? Well, their problems didn't even rate as statistically significant.

Naturally, we suggest that you get more sleep. But we know that won't always be possible. So you need to find ways to improve your *quality* of sleep, even if you can't fit in the recommended hours.

That's where GH and the incredible power of insulin come into play.

Increasing GH can make your sleep more restful even when you're not spending as much time in your slumber, according to researchers at Oregon Health and Science University. But more importantly, more GH and better sleep quality will lower cortisol, which offsets the damage caused by fewer hours of rest.

WHAT IS CORTISOL?

Cortisol is one of the power players in the hormone game. Quite simply: fuck with cortisol, and it will fuck you up. That said, cortisol isn't all bad. It's tied to your fight-or-flight response. So the occasional surge in cortisol can be helpful for everything from lifting more weight to improving your immunity and even helping brain function and memory.

But like most things in life, the poison is in the dose. Cortisol levels are oftentimes increased due to stress. And we're not just talking about watching your team blow another lead with ten seconds left in the game or dealing with a pain-in-the-ass boss. This is every type of stress, such as not sleeping enough, having too much fat on your body, or worrying about how to resolve conflict with your significant other. Even eating the wrong foods can stress your body and increase cortisol.

And when cortisol levels remained elevated or are constantly spiked, your body eventually breaks down in every way possible. You age faster. You gain weight more easily. And you suffer from disease.

So in order for you to remain happy and good-looking, it's important that you keep your cortisol in check.

You see, high cortisol creates interruptions in sleep patterns. In other words, it makes you sleep like crap and wake up feeling even worse. But it's a vicious cycle because poor rest means your cortisol becomes elevated even more, which will ensure that your sleep will continue to get worse. What's more, less sleep also robs you of your testosterone, according to a study published in the *Journal of the American Medical Association*. And we're not talking a tiny drop; the researchers indicated that poor-quality sleep could cause up to a 15 percent decrease in testosterone—giving you one more reason to focus on your rest.

What's most amazing—and scary—is that the changes were almost instant. After just one week, the researchers noted the drop in testosterone and the men reported feeling more moody, having less vigor, and struggling with concentration. Even worse, the highest drops occurred during the afternoon hours and into the late evening (around ten P.M.)—meaning your testosterone will be lowest when you need it most to perform in bed.

So while we'd love for you to get your eight hours of sleep, we'll settle for improving the quality of your rest and leaving you with plenty of time for the more important things in life like watching football, reading books, and having sex.

5. Insulin Spikes

Have you ever had a bagel and then felt like you needed a nap? Of course. We've all been there. Doesn't matter if it's bagels or pizza. Some delicious carb meals knock you down quicker than a Tyson uppercut.

A lot of nutrition "experts" will tell you that you should simply avoid bagels. But we're not going to do that because we love bagels. And there's no amount of science that will make bagels less delicious than they are. Our advice is the opposite—if you like carbs, we want you to be able to eat them. It's when you don't take the right approach that your intermittent treats can create an internal environment that is dangerous for your long-term health.

Anyone who's ever been on a low-carb diet can tell you that eating carbs crashes your insulin and makes you tired. Once in a while is not much of an issue, but the frequency with which you do this can be dangerous. If your insulin is spiking and crashing all over the place every single day, you've got a problem. You're going to cause something called insulin resistance, which is the opposite of what we want—insulin sensitivity.

With insulin resistance your insulin is chronically high, which means your body is primed for fat storage. You might not think this is your issue, but the standard American diet includes about 300 grams of carbs per day. And if you enjoy a bagel for breakfast, a sandwich for lunch, pasta for dinner, and some crackers and fruit as snacks throughout the day, then you're already near the danger zone. And that doesn't even account for sweetened drinks (that includes juice), desserts, and the "healthy" muffins they offer at work.

Even the USDA screws up its recommendations. It suggests about 200 to 300 grams of carbohydrates per day. While we're all about the occasional carb binge, it's not good to eat like this every day. And here's why: the insulin spikes will become more pronounced, and it will take less food to achieve them. It's sort of like being an alcoholic. But instead of needing more alcohol to feel drunk, you need fewer carbs to achieve the same insulin spike. This is why so many people fear carbs. When you eat too many carbs consistently, it makes each and every carbohydrate you eat worse for your body. And that's exactly what we want to avoid.

Insulin resistance isn't just inconvenient; it's downright dangerous. Obviously we're worried about fat loss and muscle. But there's also a direct relationship between insulin and failing health—including obesity and diabetes. Do you want to be fat, ugly, and diabetic? Of course not. No one does. We want you to be fit, lean, and awesome.

And that starts with establishing a smarter baseline of carbohydrate consumption. We don't want you all over the map. Not only is eating high carbs every day bad for you but so is cycling between high and low carbs consistently—that's exactly what many diet books get wrong. It's not all or none. It's about finding the sweet spot where you're still eating and enjoying carbs but not doing it at a level that drives your insulin insane. And at the same time, you want to control insulin in a way that allows you to indulge in cheat meals that will use a temporary insulin spike to improve your body and your health. We can help.

You'll see that when you time your bagels . . . or pizza . . . or ice cream correctly, you can increase your insulin sensitivity, build more muscle, and even strip off fat.

6. Lack of Confidence

Having high testosterone isn't about being an asshole. It's about not being a little bitch. (Write that down, and tweet it while you're at it.)*

Here's what we mean. Testosterone is your body's life force. It directly impacts your energy, your mood, and your drive. Low testosterone makes you less assertive. And this rears its head in all the wrong places—in your decision making, in conversations, and at work. Even when you know you're right or when you're the expert, you justify your lack of assertiveness by telling yourself that being obsequious and showing acquiescence is beneficial, that you shouldn't make waves. That's ridiculous.

In life, success is achieved by the confident, the bold, and the aggressive. No one wants to promote a little bitch. No one even wants to be around one. Having an opinion is the foundation of greatness. Followers don't become leaders and rise to the top. It's the people who are willing to voice their ideas—even when they are unusual or radical—who get heard.

Confidence is what allows you to step out of your comfort zone and take risks, whether it's speaking up at work or starting your own business or going after the girl you want. Confidence is what helps you develop the courage. If you're never willing to take a risk, you have almost no shot of building anything worth mentioning. There are no statues built of those who lived lives of mediocrity, and on the tomb of no heroes will you find the words, "He played it safe."

Lacking confidence? A boost in your natural testosterone production is what you need. More testosterone literally changes your mind-set from a physiological standpoint. You'll

---

* No, seriously: tweet that shit. And while you're at it, use the official hashtag for this book, #alphastatus.

believe in yourself. You'll have confidence. And you'll find that you have a harder time not voicing your opinions and stepping up. And that's why we're going to show you every single way to naturally elevate your testosterone levels, so you can walk through life brazenly, like an Alpha should.

7. Boobs Instead of Pecs

Listen, you produce estrogen. There's nothing wrong with it. It's a part of life. Estrogen is the yin to your testosterone's yang.

The real issue is that you're probably producing much more estrogen than you should be. And that extra estrogen can have some pretty depressing side effects. How depressing? How about man-boobs?

Men love boobs—just not on their own body.

And while we wish push-ups and bench presses would fix the problem, they won't. Trust us. They're what every guy with "moobs" is trying right now, and they're not working.

You can grow a beard or a manly mustache, but if you have moobs, it's hard to feel like a guy when you look like a chick.

In the mildest of cases, moobs are simply localized fat storage influenced by your estrogen. In the worst cases, you'll end up with something called gynecomastia. This is where your problem goes beyond fat that can be lost. With gynecomastia, it's a change in tissue. The fat attaches itself to your mammary glands and can only be removed by surgery. You obviously don't want that.

This is not meant to be depressing. It's a useful realization because you can kill the problem while it's still mild. Your fix is the training and diet that you'll find in part 3. These programs will minimize your estrogen production and boost testosterone to ward off any unwanted side effects. Combine that with dietary changes that will keep you away from estrogen-producing foods, and you'll be feeling and looking like more of a man.

8. Men Turned into Boys

The negative effects of high estrogen aren't just limited to confidence and appearance. Let's take it a step farther. A lack of testosterone or a surplus of estrogen can strongly impact your general psychological and emotional states.

The idea of being weepy, whiny, or wussy probably isn't appealing to you. And we're not talking about how you feel when you watch *Brian's Song*. (If you don't well up during that, you have no heart.) But if, like most guys, you don't have your estrogen under control, you're headed toward a life of tears.

Your high estrogen will affect you emotionally, screwing with you on every level. Joking aside, this isn't about crying at Hallmark commercials—it's about a serious hormonal imbalance that can affect things from basic decision making to depression and thoughts of suicide. In fact, according to researchers in Australia, men with low testosterone and high estrogen are *three times* more likely to suffer from depression.

9. Fertility Issues

Legacy.

As humans, procreation is one of our strongest drives. It's a point of pride: you are not only the sum of your life's work—you are also reflected by your offspring. And you directly impact and influence the lives of the humans you create.

But what if you couldn't produce children because of a problem you could easily prevent? That's the reality for any man who suffers from low testosterone.

At this point in your life, having children might not be a great concern. Or maybe you're not interested at all. But whether you have children should be a conscious decision, not one that is thrust on you by a hormonal imbalance that you could easily avoid.

Research has found that men with low testosterone are more likely to suffer from varicoceles—a medical condition in which the veins in your testicles are enlarged. While having big balls might sound like a good thing, in reality this condition is linked to infertility.

One of the reasons you could suffer from low testosterone is because you have a lack of something called luteinizing hormone. This hormone affects the production of both testosterone and sperm. While this is reversible with treatment, even temporary sterility is frighteningly serious. With hormonal adjustment, you can right the ship quickly.

BECOME THE HERO . . . NOW

We're going to go out on a limb and say that nothing we just shared sounds appealing to you. But this is just the beginning of how you've been misled by the fitness industry and why the advice you've been given is directly leading to some of the problems we mentioned. And in the next chapter, you'll learn exactly how to make sense of all the misinformation and to identify the myths that are corrupting your body and your hormones.

THE SEVEN TRAITS OF THE ALPHA

*"Leadership consists not in degrees of techniques but in traits of character . . .
and it imposes on both leader and follower alike the burdens of self-restraint."*
—LEWIS H. LAPHAM

Before you move any farther in this book, it's important that you understand what's on the table. As we've mentioned before, our goal is to completely redefine what it means to be the Alpha. We want to strip away all the negative connotations about the Alpha being cocky, the associations with meatheads, and the belief that Alphas are primarily pickup artists.

When people think of the Alpha, they generally think of someone along the lines of Fight Club's Tyler Durden, who is a quintessential embodiment of the traditional concept. Existing as the alter ego of the narrator, Tyler embodies all the best qualities that the narrator believes don't exist within him. Durden manifests himself as all the best parts but brings with him the absolute worst: he is attractive, strong, intelligent, and clever;* however, he's also destructive, anarchistic, narcissistic, and detached. While he is an exaggeration, Durden lives as what our society considers Alphas to be. He is confident, but arrogant. Self-assured, but self-involved. He is charismatic, but dangerous.

Whether or not Chuck Palahniuk (author of Fight Club) was intending to make Tyler a representation of the Alpha is not an issue; the reality is, he came pretty close to embodying the polluted idea of the Alpha. In the zeitgeist, an Alpha isn't ideal. It's completely flawed.

Society has Alphas pegged wrong; they are not the strongest guy or the one who makes the most money or has the most confidence. If you read the dictionary, the Alpha is the top of any group. He's the captain, the quarterback, the CEO of a Fortune 500 company. The Alpha is success. But more importantly, it's a persona dependent on individual progress and success. It's about attaining the highest level of self-mastery and always trying to improve.

The nutrition information, the training, and the hormonal optimization in this book—all that stuff is tremendously important. But we could have written that information like any other fitness book. We didn't do that because we have higher ambitions: we want to change minds as well as bodies. We want to change lives. And part of that is taking ownership of

---

* To be a bit more descriptive and quote Tyler on himself, he says, "All the ways you wish you could be, that's me. I look like you wanna look, I fuck like you wanna fuck, I am smart, capable, and most importantly, I am free in all the ways that you are not."

the word Alpha—reshaping it from the ground up, giving it a new definition, and adorning it with new connotations.

The first step on the path to harnessing your inner Alpha is attaining a higher level of physical prowess. That's the foundation of what we'll teach you. But from that physical transformation, other positive traits will follow, such as leadership, kindness, intelligence, and success. Throughout this book, we'll share the fundamental lessons that will help you become the Alpha who embodies and masters these traits. This is a guide that will not only show you how to become a more efficient and powerful human but also how to live a more fulfilling and prosperous life.

We understand the Alpha has some connotations that are hard to break. That's why we want to define the traits so you understand what it really means to be the Alpha. Your evolution will depend on remembering that the poison is in the dose. We've identified the traits, but ultimately the Alpha understands when to turn these traits on and off, and when pushing too far leads down a path that is harmful to you and others. We'll show you those barriers, but it's up to you to draw the line and stay the path.

■ ALPHA TRAIT #1

Helpful—But Not Condescending
The drive to become successful isn't simply a means to a narcissistic and individualistic end. The Alpha understands that taking care of his primary goals is only part of creating the life he wants; the other half is influencing and shaping the world he lives in. It's taking what you've learned—the good and the bad—and being able to pay that knowledge forward and make the world a better place. That is the foundation of this entire book: take the lessons we have learned about how to create an unreal life, combine them with your own life lessons to create your own version, and share them.

But being helpful has its limits. The Alpha gives advice and encourages others, but he does not look to do things for them. He understands that they need to do things on their own, and while they sometimes may need assistance—whether with advice or guidance— the Alpha realizes that if he were to overstep his bounds and solve the problems for them, they wouldn't learn. The Alpha doesn't micromanage the people in his life. That's not being helpful; that's being condescending. That is assuming that his own ability to solve problems supersedes that of everyone else.

Believing that you are the only one who can fix things is the height of egotism, the pro-verbial, "If you want something done right, just do it yourself." This mind-set is one of the *most damaging opinions you can have. By doing tasks for others, you're removing their ability to help themselves advance, limiting their growth potential, and imposing your will on them in a way that is not helpful but damaging.*

While being helpful is important, trying to be too helpful can go too far. If you are trying to do everything for everyone, you're not saying, "I want you to succeed." What you really mean is, "I don't think you can do it." It's an insult wrapped in a facade of kindness. The Alpha is a leader and a motivator but always in the context of letting the people you're helping blaze their own path.

That applies to us, and this book, as well. We don't think we have all the answers, but we know we have some of them. We've discovered certain traits, characteristics, and triggers that can serve as guidelines to help you master the circumstances that dictate your life. And so the purpose of this book is not to solve all your problems for you—it's to give you the tools to solve them yourself.

We'll show you the elements that will make you stronger, smarter, and more confident. These attributes will improve how you look, help you at your job, and boost your sex life— but only when you take those lessons and apply them in your own manner. Keep that in mind for everything you learn; you must apply knowledge in a way that works for you.

■ ALPHA TRAIT #2

Confident—But Not Cocky

The previous incarnation of the Alpha was always thought of as cocky. As we already stated, you know the alpha male as the guy who put others down to elevate himself. The redefined Alpha is not characterized by some overt cockiness that is projected to hide deeper insecurities but rather by a true confidence, an honest assessment of his strengths and weaknesses as well as what he can immediately achieve and what he needs to work on. The true Alpha doesn't need to put others down to feel better. His assessment of self isn't defined by a comparative analysis. It's an internal drive that fuels motivation and success.

Therefore, the Alpha elevates others to display his confidence in his ability to share thoughts, ideas, and plans that can positively influence the world around him and the people in it. If you have good ideas, you should share them. If you think you can help people, then you should take action. If you think you're the right guy for a woman, then you should prove it to her. This is what confidence enables—taking action in every form possible. But that action should never be used to denigrate another individual. When you accept who you are and appreciate who you can be, your confidence immediately becomes much more genuine, your insecurities become less potent, you create more control, and you experience more success.

■ ALPHA TRAIT #3

Vain—But Not Conceited

Listen, there should be an understanding that good-looking people can go a little farther in this world. It's not a hard-line rule, but it is a general observation that has been proven over and over again. English researchers found that men who are rated as more attractive also happen to make more money in their jobs and have higher positions. This is just a correlation, but it's not the only study that has recognized the relationship.

A little bit of vanity is a good thing because it's really just a manifestation of wanting to take care of yourself. When you look good, you feel good. When you feel good, you exude an energy that improves your world and the world of the people you interact with.

Just like extreme cockiness is the bad side of confidence, the downside of vanity is when it progresses to conceit. There is nothing wrong with wanting to be ridiculously good-looking. The problems only begin when you start believing that because you're good-looking—or more muscular or leaner or smarter or wealthier—that you're better than everyone else. That's conceit.

The Alpha understands this differentiation. He doesn't want to improve his body to be better than others. Instead, the focus is about the feelings of achievement that go along with reshaping his body. The process of self-improvement makes him feel better as a means of inspiring his confidence and building a precedent of success. As you'll find out later in the book, creating physical success is a gateway to generating success in every other aspect of your life.

The Alpha knows this and realizes that while looks or brains or money or muscles may give him an edge, they don't make him a better person. His value is determined by his actions and what he does for other people and the world.

■ ALPHA TRAIT #4

Prideful—But Not Arrogant

The difference between pride and arrogance is a fine line but one that separates those men who inspire from those considered assholes. Everything depends on how you react to your *success. Do you share your successes as a means to promote more creative and progressive thought—or do you expect things to happen because of what you've already accomplished?*

Arrogance is assuming that, because you've reached a certain level, you're entitled to certain privileges and opportunities. People who rest on their laurels are arrogant. On the other hand, pride is acknowledging your success but always retaining the mind-set of an intern. You have to earn every opportunity, hustle for every success, and prove yourself over and over again—no matter who you are and what you've done previously.

The difference between these two qualities is easily differentiated. Do you talk about your prior successes as a means to create new opportunities for yourself and others, or is it done with the expectation that people will automatically react with reverence and feel humbled in your presence? Are you looking to always work hard—on your projects or partnerships—or are you simply looking for a way to beat the system and receive what you think you should be given?

The Alpha understands that pride is an essential part of self-actualization. You can't improve yourself and the world you live in if you don't acknowledge your success. This is change psychology that depends on reinforcement. You need to believe you are good, and the only way to do that is to reference what you've done right. At the same time, pointing to prior success shouldn't change the fundamental drive to become better or the effort you put in during that process.

In the end, the difference is simple. Pride is the province of the Alpha who has done and will continue to do great things—and arrogance is the calling card of dickheads and pretenders who are simply masquerading as power players.

■ ALPHA TRAIT #5

Humble—But Not Self-Loathing

The drive to avoid arrogance can swing too far and bring you to a place where you no longer value yourself or what you achieve. Just as pride is important for acknowledging your successes, humility is equally important for confessing how hard it was to become better and accepting that you may not be the best and that you have a lot of work to do to get where you want to go.

Humility is important. It keeps us sane. It keeps us grounded. Most importantly, it keeps us hungry. Understanding that you are smart is essential to building the confidence you need to achieve; reminding yourself that you're not Einstein is a strong driver that will help you learn more and become even smarter. But thinking that because you're not Einstein means you're patently stupid, well, that goes past the point of humility and dips into self-loathing.

This dark side can manifest itself in a way that is truly self-destructive. When you become self-loathing, you venture into a universe where you are incapable of taking pride or credit for any success. Self-loathers genuinely lack so much confidence that anything that is accomplished is never seen as a direct result of their effort, time, or contributions. They are paralyzed by a belief that no matter what they do, they are not good enough. Self-loathers downplay achievements, direct praise only toward others, and castigate themselves for all shortcomings and failures. In other words, the highs are still considered valleys, and the lows can drive confidence to the depths of hell.

The Alpha understands that anyone who can't be a little self-deprecating is taking life—and himself—too seriously. He's humble and hungry, but he gives himself credit where it's due. And he never, ever loses faith in himself.

■ ALPHA TRAIT #6

Tolerant—But Not Weak

We probably don't need to tell you this, but you're going to have to put up with some crap in life. Whether it's with friends, loved ones, coworkers, or bosses, part of life is dealing with crap. It's an inevitable fact that no one can avoid. Patience and tolerance are essential to understanding your place in the world, as is being comfortable with opposing opinions and beliefs. Your opinion is not the only one that matters, and your job is not to convince everyone to see the world as you do.

Whether it's in the office or at the bar, you can't be argumentative with everything that goes against your worldview and values. You have to be tolerant of people's mistakes, shortcomings, and personal opinions. Doing otherwise is being narrow-minded and an asshole. And you don't want to be an asshole.

At the same time, there are lines in life. And if people cross them—whether repeatedly or egregiously—you have to be willing to put your foot down. This doesn't always mean being aggressively confrontational; in many situations, the Alpha displays his tolerance by addressing inappropriate behaviors with helpful solutions. In the workplace, when people are screwing up, punishing them for their mistakes is not always the best way to fix the solution. Addressing the problem and providing an alternative path to help them become better is an approach that works best for everyone.

Other times, a more aggressive approach is needed. Within the working world, you'll inevitably have a boss or superior who will go above and beyond to make your life miserable. You should feel empowered to address these behaviors in a way that improves the situation. In these moments, you need to be aggressive and confident. You need to confront the problem, lay the cards on the table, and leave your adversary with no choice but to see the situation that has been created and the steps that need to be taken. As the Alpha, you should always be thinking about solutions, not problems. And in the most extreme cases, this might mean you need to be able to walk away and find a different job.

Part of being the Alpha is understanding that the toxicity in the world around you can literally make you a less evolved person, making you more unhappy and thereby negatively impacting every related aspect of your life.

Determine your morals and values. Remind yourself that not every disagreement is a point of contention. But remember that being tolerant is not an excuse to sacrifice the core of who you are. The Alpha inspires the world around him to become better, and that can't happen if you're too fearful to voice your opinion and settle for a life where you're always the bitch.

■ *ALPHA TRAIT #7*

Dedicated—But Not Obsessed

We're all familiar with the image of the workaholic. You know him as the guy who stays late at the office and works himself to the bone. Doesn't matter if it's Monday at eleven A.M. or Saturday at two A.M.—the workaholic is a machine designed for one purpose: getting things done.

On one hand, we admire these people. There's something to be said about a great work ethic, hustle, and desire to take on seemingly impossible projects. On the other hand, there's an aspect of the workaholic that we pity. That's because there's a fine line between dedication and obsession, and knowing where to draw that line makes all the difference between whether your hustle and grit are virtuous traits or deleterious characteristics that cause you to lose sight of what's really important in your life.

The difference between dedication and obsession is that dedicated people work themselves toward a point of achievement. The Alpha outlines goals so there is a quantitative or qualitative way of determining success. This is what keeps him humble and hungry but also prevents him from endlessly chasing more work and spiraling into obsessions. The obsessed are those who can't pull themselves away from their desks. They focus infinitely on one thing and one thing only, so much so that everything else important in their life becomes blurred or diluted, or at worst disappears. The obsessed oftentimes possess another dangerous trait—being self-loathing.

In order to draw the line, the Alpha understands that being dedicated means approaching goals like a sprint, in bursts of concentrated effort. Obsession is a marathon, a life spent chained to a treadmill chasing a carrot with no hope of ever feeling satisfied—and that unfulfilled feeling laces the very essence of everything in life.

The French Renaissance writer Michel de Montaigne once wrote, "Obsession is the wellspring of genius and madness." While this is true in the sense that the top 1 percent of 1 percent of all achievements might be unlocked by only a single-minded pursuit, madness is the more common consequence of obsession. It leaves you bitter, empty, and alone. Alphas are dedicated to their families, friends, health, and most of all to themselves. They are dedicated to improvement, but they are not tied to a narcissistic view that impairs their ability to create a rich, multifaceted existence.

CHAPTER 2

Choose Your Own Adventure

ACCEPTING YOUR ROLE AS THE HERO

*"There is one rule, above all others, for being a man.
Whatever comes, face it on your feet."*

—ROBERT JORDAN, *THE GREAT HUNT*

ARIA CASINO, LAS VEGAS

"**The reason every guy struggles with fitness** can be explained by Joseph Campbell. Understand that, and the transformation becomes easier."

The man across from me glanced down at the cards on the table, his eyes lingering just a second too long on the eight of spades, which was the far right in the line. The eight had come on the turn and had been preceded on the flop by the queen of hearts, ten of diamonds, and ace of diamonds. He reached into his stack and tossed some chips in the middle. I wasn't sure how much—*some chips* was the best description, since he didn't make a verbal declaration, or even take the time to count out a bet. Just grab and bet. In poker, this is generally either a very strong move or a very weak one; it all depends on the man making it.

I was sitting in the poker room at the Aria Casino, Adam Bornstein on my left. Adam was finally taking a break from questioning me long enough to let me assess my next move. The guy across the table, the one who had made the bet, sat in stony silence as well. I didn't know his name, but I mentally labeled him Trucker Hat, for the very obvious reason that, contrary to all logic, he was still wearing a trucker hat about five years after society had collectively decided that it was no longer okay to do so.

It was 12:47 A.M. in Vegas, but my body was still on New York time, and I had been playing for a few hours already. I should have been exhausted, but instead felt elated. It was too early for Trucker Hat to be making moves like this.

I glanced briefly at my cards, as though they might have changed in the last minute or so. Didn't matter. Play the man, not the cards. I counted out a pile of chips from my stack, and set it aside. I took a few deep breaths, deep enough for Trucker Hat to see. I stared at the queen, then the ace. I waited a bit longer and then doubled, declaring a raise. Eleven black chips went into the pot.

"You really think that'll work?" Adam resumed his questioning once the chips were down. It was a game within a game.

I glanced at Adam, then at Trucker Hat. "Raising? Yeah, usually does. Makes guys think twice about calling with middle pair." I ended the speech with a smirk and a wink. Adam wasn't talking about the bet. I knew that.

"What? No," Adam said. "*Campbell*. Do you think guys will get Campbell? Not everyone's a fucking *Star Wars* geek."

His point was lost on me. I don't understand people who don't like *Star Wars*.

"Dude, *everyone* gets Campbell. It doesn't matter if they haven't read his stuff. That's the entire point. It's burned into the consciousness of every culture. It's the way we tell stories. The monomyth isn't . . . isn't fucking *invalidated* because you don't know about it—it's the fact that you can understand it without learning it that makes it *more* valid. And valuable. I think they'll get it."

Trucker Hat was eyeing me. Well, sometimes. His eyes darted back and forth from my face to Adam's to my chips and back to me. He was clearly trying to reconcile the spectacle of muscular guy in an unnecessarily tight T-shirt* talking about Campbell. In the mind of most people, meatheads and myths are probably not related.

Adam considered my words. Trucker Hat considered his move. I considered his chips. Call.

STARTING FROM SCRATCH

Who the hell is Joseph Campbell? And what happened with the bet?

If you are like most people, after reading that your brain is probably processing one of those two thoughts; possibly both.

Why? It's something called *anterograde memory*. We focus on the last thing we heard and forget about everything else that preceded it. Our memories therefore, are the result of strategic timing of information that is shared—or not shared. Knowing this, it's easy to

* Hey, if a fat guy who isn't a trucker can wear a trucker hat, I can wear a shirt one size too small. Focus on the story, okay? —JR

understand how most people come to understand the world. It's always about who has the final word. And when it comes to your body and health, the wrong people are repeatedly delivering the final salvo that leads you down a frustrating path. It's the same path you take with every diet and fitness book.

Which is why we arrived at Campbell. It's time to take a new path and an entirely new approach to your life and your body. This is bigger than a fitness book. This is a life overhaul. And Campbell's ability to make it blatantly clear how we subconsciously avoid or fail to recognize the hurdles that prevent us from becoming who we want to be was the perfect structure to help us end your frustration and guide you to a better life—to take you from ordinary man to Alpha.

CHARTING A NEW COURSE: THE HERO'S JOURNEY

Joseph Campbell was an American writer and lecturer who was best known for his discussions of mythology—particularly comparative mythology. He examined the myths across cultures, generations, and centuries, and he realized that all great stories converged around analogous concepts. Campbell plotted an outline that covered the universal patterns that appear in myths from the cultures of antiquity like Greece, Sumer, and Babylon; medieval and Renaissance-age folklore from Germany, Spain, and Britain; and even more modern stories in books that were published through the mid-twentieth century. This pattern results in a seventeen-stage storytelling structure known as the monomyth.

Also known as the Hero's Journey, the monomyth was covered in Campbell's definitive work, *The Hero with a Thousand Faces.* This book became one of the most influential of the twentieth century and introduced the masses to the concept that all great heroes have similar paths.

Taking it a step farther, writers in other disciplines have applied the monomyth to everything from psychological treatment to athletic programs—all with equal success. Campbell's theories can be applied to nearly any concept, and will prove suitable for examination of any great change. The monomyth is universal, and the journey exists in the lives of all men—you, me, your buddies at the bar—and not just the characters in the books you read and the movies you watch.

The problem: we fail to realize that we are the hero and that our life should be a tale worth telling.

This is why we oftentimes don't reach our potential—because we completely avoid the opportunity to take the journey that can improve our lives. This is important for one simple reason: you *need* to believe you can change your life. This is the very foundation of behavioral change psychology and the determining factor of whether the information you receive in this book will actually help you.

People *want* to change and become better, but when they don't believe they can, they end up stuck in the same place: the first stage of the Hero's Journey—the Ordinary World.

According to Campbell, the Ordinary World is the boring and mundane existence where the hero lives at the beginning of his journey. It marks the sharpest contrast from the Special World where the hero eventually ends up.

The Ordinary World is Luke's farm in *Star Wars*. It's Dorothy's farm in *The Wizard of Oz*. It's the Joads' farm in *The Grapes of Wrath*.* But it's also your desk. Really, it's any farm. Ever. It's your desk. It's your couch. It's your bedroom. It's the office parties you hate going to. It's the food that makes you feel like shit. It's every fitness book you've ever read.

Most people just accept this. They swallow their reality as the only one that's possible. It's normal. It happens. But it doesn't have to be that way.

THE EVOLUTION OF AVERAGE

If you consider—as we do—that every great change you make in your life is an adventure, then the starting point for your journey is *your* Ordinary World. It's a world that you know, whether it's tame and sane or chaotic and destructive. However, it's a world you also want to leave. That's why you have this book. If you were happy with where you are, you would not seek change; if on some level you didn't crave that change, you would not be reading these words right now.

But it's good that you are—because change is exactly what *Engineering the Alpha* is about.

We want this book to do more for you than just help you get in shape.

Don't get us wrong. We're happy to pack ten pounds of muscle onto your body, drop you to less than 10 percent fat, and make your sex life almost too much to handle. And these changes will happen. We'll teach you why optimizing your hormones is the key to everything, and we'll share the science and real world results that make this an undeniable truth.

But more than anything, we want this book to serve as a blueprint and a guide to creating your own version of the Hero's Journey. Remember, the goal of all of this is to engineer you into the Alpha version of *you*. And in order for that to happen, you must reach a moment of Apotheosis—one of the late stages of the Hero's Journey—which is when you achieve, even if only for a second, the highest level of self-awareness.

Remember, these things don't just apply to mythology; this is an essential psychological process that you need to go through in order to reach your goals, and apotheosis is one of the most important steps in that process. It's the moment when you become who you were meant to be.

---

* Man, what is it with farms? If you live on a farm, consider yourself lucky, because you're probably going to go on some life-changing adventure to save the world.

Your hormones make these improvements possible, but the biggest hurdle is learning how to navigate the journey and not fall victim to the traps and barriers that sidetrack the ordinary man.

By avoiding those, you'll unlock your truest and highest levels of potential. And when that happens, no dream scenario—whether it's for your career, your body, or your personal life—will be untouchable.

But none of this is possible until you realize that you need to pave your own path and stop jumping around from one program to another, taking an ADD approach to changing your life from the inside out. You need to go *big*. Invest in your search for the truth and play out your hand with confidence so that you can see what happens when you make a gamble on the only investment that always pays out: yourself.

BACK TO THE GAME: ARE YOU ALL IN?

The pot was now at just under three grand. Could be a good haul. But now that Adam had brought me back into the debate, I was focused on Campbell.

"I think," I began, just as the dealer laid out the next card, "it's relatable if you explain it correctly. It's not just about myths. It's about being a hero, being more than you are. Evolving. It's about—"

"Becoming the Alpha," Adam finished with a smile. "It's to you, by the way."

The action was to me, that is. Another card had appeared on the board; Trucker Hat had checked, passing the action.

I watched him, sitting in a state of anticipation and self-satisfaction. It's funny, sometimes, watching people. You learn a lot at a poker table. I glanced down at the final card to have hit the board—a two of hearts. It didn't change anything.

Shrugging, I pushed my remaining chips toward the center of the table, totaling $6,680. "All in." Sometimes you have to give them what they want.

Trucker Hat jumped out of his chair and called, pushing his chips in without hesitation. In poker, this is known as snapcalling or instacalling. His chips brought the pot to $10,300ish.

Adam took a deep breath and asked, "So what part of the Hero's Journey are we at right now?"

"This would be the Ordeal—the climax, the big showdown. The lightsaber battle on the Death Star. Stage eight, I believe."

"I was kidding. Only you could think about the monomyth with 10K on the line," said Adam with a chuckle.

Trucker Hat turned over his cards to show two eights. "I got a set of eights," he declared triumphantly. Strong hand.

I looked at Trucker Hat, then at Adam. "Apotheosis."

Turning over my cards to show a jack and a nine, completing a straight. I had the nuts, or the best possible hand.* Trucker Hat was not pleased. Adam was.

"Apotheosis, huh?"

"Yeah. That's stage nine, a moment of enlightenment or inspiration. Now, on to stage ten. Time to put this money to some good use. Let's grab a steak."

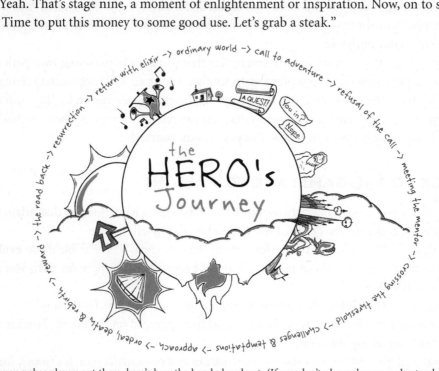

* For you poker players out there, here's how the hand played out. (If you don't play poker or understand poker terminology, this may be lost on you.) We were sitting 5/10 No Limit Hold'em (NL for the truly initiated) at the Aria, which has a $3,000 cap on the buy-in. Adam was in an empty seat at the table but wasn't playing; he'd never seen someone play at those stakes and was just watching. At the start of the hand, I had about $8,200. Trucker Hat had just around $6K and was in middle position, and he made a raise to $120 in a limped pot (at that point, $60). I had J9s in the cutoff and had played a few hands with him; I assumed he was just making a move, so I raised to $380, looking to take down the pot. I was surprised when he called (bringing the pot to $820), so I figured he could have woken up with a hand. In his range, I thought anywhere from a small pocket pair to AJ or something similar (he would have popped it with AK). The flop came Qh, Td, Ad. He led out for $300, which was small for the pot. It seemed like a feeler bet, and at this point, I was putting him on an under pair since I'd seen him check-raise with top pair three times. I thought about raising but decided to just flat call (pot now $1,420) to make a huge bet on the turn. (Yes, I'm crazy like that, and I will bet $2,000 with nothing but air. If you ever play with me, you should call.) I certainly wasn't expecting to hit my gut draw, but I did. Turn comes 8s, as noted above, and I saw him come alive in his chair. At that point, my read told me the only possibilities were a set of eights or something like 9–7, meaning he now had an up-and-down draw. At this point, there were also two spades on the board, so he *could* have had a flush draw, but that was very unlikely, given that I was holding two spades. It was even more unlikely that, if he had spades, he was going to have a higher flush (I couldn't give him credit for Qs, since he would have played a pair of queens differently. And if he had Ks, he was getting all my chips). The set seemed most likely to me. I had the nut straight with a redraw to the jack-high flush. He bet some chips—which, as it turned out, was about $500. I made it $1,100, and he called, bringing the pot to $3,620. The river came 2h, making me the winner. Yay, me. I pushed for my remaining $6,680, bringing the pot to $10,300. He called for his remaining chips, and I scooped a $13K pot.

ENGINEERING THE ALPHA

SUBJECT: *Ian Estabrook*

THE ORDINARY WORLD

At the start of my transformation, I weighed 206 pounds and was a little over 15 percent body fat (measured via calipers). I was one of those guys that looked fit, but really had much to be desired. I wanted more from my body and life, but wasn't sure if I could actually reach the levels of success I imagined.

ACCEPTING THE CALL

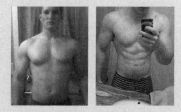

When someone is thinking of finding a mentor or hiring a coach, they usually consider the cost, and then review a list of their success stories, philosophies on training and nutrition, and training certifications. In my search for a coach, I kept all of these qualities in mind, but I was also looking for something more: "How will this person improve my quality of life?" It takes a special flair to make changes that dramatic. I did my research and stumbled upon Roman's blog. I read every blog post, and I knew I had found my coach. John Romaniello fit the bill perfectly and would be the guy to offer something different— new ideas and results.

ALPHA STATUS

After the program, my body weight dropped as low as 192 pounds at 8 percent body fat. Once I had "reset" my body, Roman geared my training toward gaining muscle mass. To my amazement, I ended my transformation weighing 206 pounds and still 8 percent body fat. This is the biggest and leanest I have ever been simultaneously, hands down. Despite not being my primary goal, Roman also got me much, much stronger.

It's hard to put into perspective how much Roman has done for me with his program. He freed me from the confines of conventional thinking and broadened my training horizons by encouraging me to not always follow the most worn path. I'll never look at training or eating the same way again, and that's a great thing. Roman's selflessness, dedication, and attention to detail has done more than just change my body—it's changed my life.

CHAPTER 3

The Truth About the Truth

BREAKING BARRIERS, AVOIDING STAGNATION, AND THE FORCES ALLIED AGAINST YOU

"The most useful piece of learning for the uses of life is to unlearn what is untrue."

—ANTISTHENES, GREEK PHILOSOPHER OF ATHENS, DISCIPLE OF SOCRATES, 445–365 BC

Here's the question every guy should be asking right now: When I try to change my body, why am I so often stuck with the same results no matter what I do?

The answer is that you have two powerful factors working against you: misinformation and a lack of focus. So we created this book to solve both problems. While you can certainly find some good information from other resources, there's also a lot of double-talk out there. Trust us—we've had to sift through it for the past decade.

But here's the thing: all of the best information is in here. And your ability to abandon all your previous frustration and confusion and leave it in the past can occur if you take one simple step—you leave the Ordinary World.

Your Ordinary World, like any that Campbell has written about, is not comfortable, but it is familiar. Stepping outside of it and rejecting what everyone else is doing is scary, but staying in it should be even scarier.

As with any hero who sees the promise of stepping beyond the Threshold, once you have seen the potential for something greater—what is captured by Campbell in mythic structure and known as the Special World—you should be unwilling to settle for something less than what is possible.

If you are tempted to read on and make changes—then this book, these words, and these pages will drive you to a life-changing experience. If you've learned anything, it's that you know your life could be better.

To paraphrase Campbell, we believe that all men were meant to be heroes of their own tale. To go a bit beyond him, we also believe that men should *look* and *act* like heroes: that they should look strong and be confident, look great and be great.

But in order to get there, you need to take the next step in the journey. And if you cannot bear the thought of *not* taking that step, then you have heard—as all heroes do—the most important sound a man can ever hear: the Call to Adventure.

RING . . . RING . . .

The hardest part about this entire book won't be the workouts, the diet, or finding a way to make time for all the sex you'll be having. It's going to be letting go of ideas that you "know" are facts. After all, in order to make room for what is right, you must first purge what is wrong.

Like a quarterback learning a new playbook, you have to forget your old coaches and dissociate yourself from much of what you have been led to believe is true. And therefore your assessment of any situation is filtered through the lens of those truths. But if those truths are not accurate, then every piece of information is being filtered through a fractured lens.

The problem is magnified when you consider the way information is shared and made viral. You know the headlines we're talking about: "The Truth About . . ." is one of the most powerful headlines possible because it incites the fear of deception. No one likes to be deceived, and fear is an extremely powerful motivator. But it's a power that is often misused and abused.

One nugget of mistruth can spread so fast that the sheer number of people who support the so-called truth strengthens the inaccuracy of claims. You see this happen at every level of life—from the playground in elementary school to the political debates in D.C. This is how myths are perpetuated, and it's a process that's difficult to overcome.

Health content is one of the worst offenders. Whether it's the same crap you read last year or the "secret" you already know, nothing is really new. Nothing feels like it's going to change your life. And most of the so-called adventures you take are circular, leading you right back to where you started—only you're now in a worse position because you're more pissed off than you were six weeks before. And you still don't have abs.

So we reviewed as much diet and fitness information as humanly possible. And through it all—the successes and the failures, the classes and the lectures, the books and journals, the clients and the mentors—we kept coming back to the same conclusion: hormones are the key to everything. And we know this because when we tested programs designed to optimize hormones, participants lost fat, built muscle, and became the heroes of their own lives.

But their success—and your success—isn't just about doing a workout or eating certain foods. It starts with something much harder: rejecting everything that the vast majority of people believe is true.

Why? Because that's what Alphas do.

This is the real secret that will allow you to follow the workouts confidently, eat with freedom, and optimize your hormones in a way that will make everything much easier. After all, that's the point of this book: to make looking great, feeling great, and living a better life easier than it has ever been.

ANSWER THE CALL

If you want to accept our information as your new reality, then you must reject your old approach.

We're telling you this because we know how you're going to react to the truths we share. Some may sound crazy. Some might not make sense. And some might sound so difficult that you'll be angry. Trust us—nothing is too hard. It's just different.

You're going to have a moment when you say, "This is bullshit." So much of what you're going to read is going to sound antithetical to what you believe and counter to what everyone else is saying. One way to reconcile what you are reading and what you want to believe is to say that we're wrong.

In the context of mythic structure, this is known as Refusing the Call. One of the earliest stages of the Hero's Journey, this is the moment when the hero is approached with the idea of the adventure itself. After he has been called, he must decide whether he should embark on his journey. In many cases, the hero may refuse—or, at least, consider refusing—the Call to Adventure.

Refusing the call is normal and extremely common, but it doesn't get you out of the Ordinary World, which is why we want to make sure you recognize the signs that could easily sabotage your journey without you even realizing it.

With traditional heroes, the refusal of the call may happen because of a sense of obligation, fear, inadequacy, or duty to family or a loved one. In the case of modern man who is seeking to become the Alpha (that's you), refusal stems from the fear of inadequacy.

Within every man lives the anxiety that he may not be able to complete the journey. And as a result, he refuses to take the first step.

Our goal is to provide you with enough evidence to rid you of fear and give you the confidence to move forward on this journey. But be warned, heroes who refuse the call are often met with consequences. As you'll see, failure to step out of your Ordinary World can lead to catastrophic health changes that will lessen the value and enjoyment of your life.

By accepting the call, you spark a form of mental rebirth: it's the death of your former beliefs, your former self, and the first step into a larger world.

Sounds deep—but isn't this what you're looking for? Because what we're offering is a new body, a new life, and something better than what you've always had.

YOU DON'T KNOW WHAT YOU DON'T KNOW

Guys aren't great when it comes to talking about emotions and feelings. Which is why we'll admit something important and vital to this program: change isn't easy. The act of change isn't some simple process of just shifting behaviors. There are psychological barriers that are connected to every change you ever make, which makes it harder for you to follow through with your intentions. And the more dramatic the changes, the more intense the psychological push to revert back to your previous tactics.

Consider this script; it'll probably sound familiar to you. Here's what happens when most guys start a new workout and diet. When they receive the new program, they start out excited. But after the initial excitement wears off, they inevitably make slight adjustments and only do the exercises they're good at. It can be something small, like doing a seated shoulder press instead of a standing barbell military press. That's just how men are programmed.

These *seem* like small, inconsequential decisions, but these changes are really just the first step toward failure.

So why does this happen? Because you haven't had the benefit of knowing the specific decisions that were separating you from Alpha status. In the best case, guys realize there's something preventing them from the pinnacle of their development. But in most cases, guys don't know that at all. They don't even realize that they have the potential to be something more than what they are. They don't realize that there is a way to get there. And they certainly don't know how to go about it.

Here's the funny thing: men's frustrations are almost universally the same. And that's because they are all still playing in the Ordinary World. It's time to leave for a new game.

LIES, MYTHS, AND WHY MEN ARE FAT

If we are to engineer the Alpha, we must take steps. And the first of those steps is to discard old beliefs. And the best way to do that is to find a consistent approach and to discard the fallacies. You need to drown out the noise.

We realize that it's not as easy as it sounds. You have half of the experts saying one thing and the other half saying something else. Case in point: You have the vegans saying that you shouldn't eat any animal product whatsoever. On the other hand, you have the paleo people saying that the key to a long and healthy life is feasting on the tasty flesh of dead creatures on a daily basis. The result: you're left really confused and inevitably trying a little bit of everything . . . and only getting fatter and more unhealthy each year.

All these disparate beliefs cause confusion. So to make it easier, we're going to outline the three steps you *need* to follow to make it realistic for you to stay on one plan and one track.

1. Cut through the noise so you can answer the call. Remember, there's a strong psychological component involved in change, so you need to buy in.

2. Learn the truth. Once you *know* that there are reasons for your prior failures (the mistruths), then we'll teach you how hormone optimization will turn you into the Alpha and transform your life.

3. Do the work. We'll supply the workout and diet programs that will serve as your vehicle to take you to the life you want.

Now that you're ready to begin the process, it's time to address all the mistruths that previously made it much harder for you to get from point A to point B. Answer this call and you'll have taken the biggest and most important step toward the successful completion of your journey. Now let's dig in to all those mistruths.

REJECT THIS THOUGHT:
Breakfast is the most important meal of the day.

For years we've been told breakfast is the most important meal of the day. In fact, you've probably been instructed by your physician not to skip breakfast—especially if you want to lose weight.

The problem? Despite the fact that roughly 90 percent of Americans eat breakfast, according to a survey conducted by the NPD group, close to 35 percent of Americans are either overweight or obese, says the Centers for Disease Control and Prevention. If eating breakfast is the solution to weight loss, then something is wrong or missing from the equation.

Before we go on, let's make sure we're on the same page. There is nothing wrong with eating breakfast. You can eat breakfast and be perfectly healthy and use it as part of an effective weight-loss plan. But breakfast is not the weight-loss elixir that it's promoted as. You see, eating first thing in the morning after you sleep actually shuts down the hormones that control your fat loss.

The problem with a traditional breakfast is that it creates a big eating window. That is, the number of hours during the day that you are consuming food. This is typically about a fifteen-hour period (between seven A.M. and ten P.M.). In a recent groundbreaking study by the scientists at the Salk Institute for Biological Studies, it was found that a larger eating window was associated with more fat storage and a higher likelihood of health problems such as diabetes and liver disease.

This study was done with mice, but the findings are too important to overlook. The mice were put on a high-fat diet that would typically cause obesity. One group of mice ate whenever they wanted, and the other could only eat for eight hours, starting in the afternoon and finishing at night. The mice that ate whenever they wanted gained fat, developed high cholesterol, high blood glucose, and liver damage. The mice with the eight-hour feeding period starting in the afternoon? They weighed 28 percent less and had no health problems, even though they ate the same amount of fatty foods.

The scientists believe that by cutting down how long you have to eat, your body does a better job of metabolizing your fat, glucose, and cholesterol. What's more, because you're eating for a smaller window of time *and* starting later in the day, your body is burning more fat. Why? Because you pushed back breakfast, extended your overnight fast (which occurs while you sleep), and became a fat-burning machine.*

What's more, by skipping breakfast (or just starting it later in the day), you also prime your body to feel hungrier less often. That's because the moment you start eating food, your body creates an expectation for calories. And for most people, that expectation means hunger pangs that are too hard to overcome, leaving you grabbing for snacks by ten A.M. and eating more calories than you should by the end of the day.

But aren't you supposed to eat more frequently? Not exactly . . .

REJECT THIS THOUGHT:
Eating frequently stokes your metabolism.

Guy walks into a gym. Meets with a trainer. Gets pitched a $600 training package. One thing leads to another and the trainer starts talking about nutrition.

"Bro, you got to eat six meals a day if you really want to lose fat. It keeps your metabolism going. You gotta keep the fire burning. That way, you can actually eat more and lose fat. It's pretty sweet, bro. It's what I do, and I'm *shrippped*!"

Forgive us for buying into the trend of demonizing the word *bro* (which we love), but some version of this happens every single day. To be fair, it's not just trainers, and the

---

* Dig in, science nerds, you're going to love this. When you fast, your body has several functions. We're going to cover this through the book in great detail. One of the most awesome of these functions is related to burning fat. When you fast, your liver produces enzymes that transform cholesterol into bile. That bile—as nasty as it sounds—is a good thing because it fires up brown fat, which is a good fat that turns the extra calories in your body into energy that you burn. It's why fasting burns fat.

people offering this advice are trying to be helpful. But they are misinformed, so let's say this as clearly and concisely as we can: eating six meals per day *does not* help you burn more fat.

Read that again, and then read it once more. Then read it out loud and watch the reactions of the people around you. They will probably look at you like you have three heads. Because everyone and their mothers (including our mothers—until we taught them) think that eating small meals helps you burn more fat, build more muscle, and fight off hunger.

Unfortunately for them, that's complete and total bullshit.

Remember when we told you that in order to come with us on your journey you have to unlearn what you have learned? To forget what you thought was true? This is one of those times.

If it's not true, then why does everyone—and we mean everyone—tell you to do this? Unfortunately, there's no good reason. We know that when you eat, you burn calories. So about thirty years ago, it was determined that if you eat more frequently you must burn more calories.

The idea seemed great. You get to eat more often and still have a lean, hard body.

But then some geniuses in white lab coats (call them scientists, doctors, professors) decided to actually test the theory. The results? Not so good for people who believe in the six-meal god.

French researchers found that there is "no evidence of improved weight loss" by eating more frequently. And they even went a step farther to show that in terms of the number of calories you burn per day, it does not matter if you graze or gorge—assuming that you're eating the number of calories you need to lose weight. So if you're told to eat 2,000 calories per day, it doesn't matter if it's separated into five 400-calorie meals or two 1,000-calorie feasts. (However, the composition of those meals does matter.)

But that's not all. Canadian researchers decided to compare three meals per day to six meals per day, breaking the six into three main meals and three snacks (the routine that has been advocated by every diet book written in the last twenty years). The results? There was no significant difference in weight loss, but the people who ate three meals per day were more satisfied and felt less hunger.

That's why on our plan we take a more realistic approach to your eating habits. It's our opinion that fewer meals per day work better for most guys. But the only rule that really matters is how much time you spend eating during the day. So we'll provide you with easy-to-follow guidelines that put you in charge of your diet within the parameters of the plan. You'll know exactly how many hours you have to eat during the day (don't worry, you have more than enough time to chow), and then you can choose how many meals you want to have within that eating period.

It's the best of both worlds. A diet plan backed by science and optimized for your goals, but without the stress of being forced to eat in a way that isn't natural to your own preferences.

REJECT THIS THOUGHT:
Your body can only digest 30 grams of protein.

A little knowledge can do a lot of damage. Several years ago a very smart researcher named Douglas Paddon-Jones ran an experiment. The design was innocent enough: test out how to maximize muscle protein synthesis. You might recognize this as your body's ability to convert protein into muscle.

Paddon-Jones found, once again, that protein builds muscle.

But he also discovered one other interesting fact. In his research, he determined that 30 grams of protein creates the same amount of maximum muscle protein synthesis as you'd receive from a 90-gram dosage. The simple conclusion—your body can't handle more than 30 grams of protein.

This was widely accepted and embraced. And suddenly a nation of men stopped eating large steaks and went back to only one scoop of protein powder in their post-workout shake. Sure, maybe it's a little more economical—but is it better for your body?

Using the same logic as the protein study, if you had sex just once in an hour and your level of arousal was the same as having sex ten times in an hour, then one bout of sex would be the same experience, right?

If you said yes, well, we don't know what to say to you.

The point we're making is this: while we have some evidence—and that evidence is not completely foolproof—that protein synthesis tops out at 30 grams, that doesn't mean you don't receive other benefits from eating more. Or that there is any harm in eating more. In fact, we know that eating a high-protein diet helps you build more muscle, stay fuller longer, and even burn more fat because protein is more metabolically active in your body (meaning it takes more calories to break down protein in your digestive system and use it as energy).

There's also a lot to be said about the pure enjoyment of things, which in this case means eating. Even if we accept Paddon-Jones's conclusions that "the body" can only utilize 30 grams of protein in "a sitting," does that mean that we shouldn't eat a porterhouse that has 60 grams of protein? Absolutely not. Porterhouse steaks are delicious. And the calories in the steak—if not the protein—will still be used in the muscle-building process.

Secondly, you'll notice that we put "the body" in quotes. Paddon-Jones's experiment was conducted with a relatively small sample size, just thirty-four people, which is important because people react to protein in different ways. So while 30 grams is a good jumping-off point, it's not the complete picture. We know that testosterone can increase protein synthesis and nitrogen retention. Meaning, if you increase testosterone—as we'll teach you throughout this book—then you can increase protein synthesis and make even better use of the protein you eat.

You'll also notice that we put "a sitting" in quotes. What constitutes a sitting? Is it thirty minutes? Sixty minutes? Obviously, we need to take into account the rate of digestion. You see, 30 grams of protein coming from the porterhouse would be broken down much more slowly than 30 grams of protein from whey hydrolysate—the fastest-digesting form for protein. So even if we could define a sitting, the type of protein would obviously factor in to the digesting.

For our purposes, it is better to look at the total amount of protein consumed in a day rather than a sitting. If you assume you can only eat 30 grams of protein at one meal and you're expected to eat 250 grams of protein in a day, you'd have no choice but to eat all of that protein in multiple meals.

But there's enough research, as we shared above, to prove that the multiple-meal hypothesis is false. And there's a mountain of evidence suggesting that your body can, in fact, digest much more than 30 grams of protein. In a study published in the *Journal of Nutrition,* scientists found no difference between eating roughly 80 percent of your protein in one meal versus four meals spread throughout the day. And by no difference, we mean that muscle gain and fat loss, as well as protein absorption, were even. And in that study, that meant that subjects were eating 54 grams of protein in one serving—or nearly double what you've been told your body can handle.

But that's not even the entire story. In that same study, only females were tested. So why should you care? As we already mentioned, the amount of muscle you have has a direct relationship to how much protein you can handle, as does the amount of testosterone in your body. And since men have more muscle and testosterone than women do, the scientists speculated that men could take in even more protein than what was discovered in the study.

Not to bore you with more science, but in another study in the *American Journal of Clinical Nutrition,* researchers found that body composition improved (less fat and more muscle) when men ate just one meal per day consisting of roughly 85 grams of protein as opposed to the same amount of protein spread across meals and more hours.

We share the science for a few reasons. First, we want you to be able to eat more protein. Guys love eating, and guys *really* love eating more protein. But you need to know that there is no drawback to eating more than 30 grams and no reason to create some imaginary cutoff. In fact, there might be a great benefit in pushing the limited findings of what our favorite scientists might recommend.

As for the exact number? Don't worry—we've done enough experiments to know what will work for your body, on this plan, with our diet and exercise design. And we will share that with you starting in chapter 8.

We love Ryan Reynolds. We've never met him, but he seems like an awesome guy, a dude who's got it all figured out. He has a movie career where he gets paid millions of dollars to play himself in every role, and he's had sex with Scarlett Johansson *and* Blake Lively. In other words, his life is pretty damn awesome.

If all of that weren't enough, Reynolds walks around shredded year-round—a difficult feat for anyone to accomplish.

Despite all that, he's not your best guy for nutritional advice, and that's why we're calling him out. You see, Mr. Reynolds—whether he realizes it or not—is one of the reasons why guys think it's bad to eat after seven P.M. When Reynolds dropped to about 5 percent body fat for his supporting role in *Blade: Trinity,* his body instantly became the new prototype and even earned him a nod for *People*'s Most Eligible Bachelor. Good for him. Bad for you.

Eating late at night is actually one of the best things you can do for your body. For starters, let's not forget the most basic of laws—and that is the first law of thermogenesis. That is, your weight is dependent on how many calories you eat (energy in) compared to how many calories you burn (energy out). While the foods you eat are very important, calories are still calories. To quote renowned nutritionist Alan Aragon, "Your body doesn't store fat more readily during the evening than any other point during the day."

What's funny is we've known this for a while. All the way back in 1987, Italian researchers compared eating earlier in the day (ten A.M.) to eating later in the day (six P.M.). In that study, there was no difference in weight loss, but fat burning was higher in the people who ate their meals after six P.M.

Several follow-up studies concluded the same thing—timing doesn't matter. And then in 2006, researchers from the University of Oregon made this bold statement: eating too many calories causes weight gain regardless of when you eat them. In other words, the timing of your meals doesn't matter. All that matters is the foods you eat.

So why not eat more calories at night? It's easier, and it makes more sense. Do you have more breakfast meetings or more dinner parties? Do you prefer drinks at night or in the morning? Eating at night is an essential component of the social fabric of our society. And living in a world where you can't eat at night and can't enjoy food with your friends and family is dumb and restrictive. And it's a reason why so many people hate dieting.

So just stop. In our diet, we're going to encourage that you eat more at night and enjoy. Your body will look better for it, you won't wake up hungry every morning, and you'll have less stress planning your day.

REJECT THIS THOUGHT:
Eat your carbs earlier in the day.

So if we're telling you it's okay to eat at night, we just mean protein, right? Cottage cheese and peanut butter—the old bodybuilder standbys. There's no possible way it's okay to eat carbs before bed.

Right?

Wrong.

In fact, eating carbs during a late-night feast might be one of the best ways to blast away your gut. Having carbs at night can cause you to release more growth hormone (GH) when you sleep. You might not know much about GH—yet—but we can tell you that it allows you to build muscle while keeping you lean. Oftentimes antiaging clinics prescribe expensive doses of GH to men looking to keep their edge. But how much better would it be to have the same impact by eating carbs at night? If you believe science and physics, that's a reality. So much so that when Israeli researchers compared people who ate their carbs in the morning with those who ate them at night, the nighttime carb feasters lost more fat and experienced less hunger.

The benefits don't end there. If you train in the morning or afternoon, consuming your carbs at night has a carryover effect toward your training. That's because those nighttime carbs will fill up your glycogen, which is the energy you need to train hard. That energy will then be utilized for your workout, but without that sick feeling you get from training just after eating.

No upset stomach, better training results, and you can have pasta for dinner? Yes, it's all true, and it's exactly what we'll prescribe as part of the diet in this book.

REJECT THIS THOUGHT:
Cardio is the best fat-loss strategy.

We don't know how we even need to address this, but somehow there is a large majority of people that believe cardio—such as long-distance running, biking, or even a slow walk on the treadmill—is the key to fat loss. Running is still the most popular physical activity, and the most common reason people run is to lose weight.

The reason the myth that cardio burns the most fat has persisted is that it's still an extremely common prescription made by doctors and fitness professionals. But cardio should never be your first line of defense against fat; slogging away on the pavement or treadmill for sixty to ninety minutes is not the key to a lean, athletic physique.

You know how we know this? Because every single fitness blogger in the world has done the same damn blog post with the same damn picture comparing the sprinter to the marathon runner. In it, the sprinter looks jacked, lean, and muscular, while the marathon runner looks gangly, ill, and thin.

The point that they're making is that long-duration cardio may be good for weight reduction, but it's not ideal for a great-looking body. Science shows us that all exercise burns calories, but all activity is not created equal. The low-intensity, long-duration cardio might help you drop weight, but a significant percentage of that might be muscle. Whereas weight training or high-intensity work (whether with resistance-training exercises or sprints) will ensure that the majority of calories you burn are fat. More importantly, it'll build and maintain your muscle, which will help your metabolism continue burning calories for twenty-four to forty-eight hours and improve your insulin levels so the food you eat is not as readily stored as fat.

REJECT THIS THOUGHT:
Light weights + high reps = shredded body

Math equations suck—especially those that don't actually end with the correct solution. The equation you see above is one of the most commonly believed in the fitness world. And yet, despite millions of people pumping away for endless reps, we still don't have a nation of Roman warriors (no pun intended . . . okay, maybe a little).*

Would you be surprised if we told you there's nothing inherently beneficial about high reps and low weights? Probably not. If you just do lots of light-weight reps and there's no struggle, your body won't change. Likewise, if you follow a traditional bodybuilder approach, with lots of sets and rest, then you won't create a metabolic change.

With light weights, not only are you *not* lifting enough weight to cause growth, but also your workout is not designed to burn fat. You're not really challenging yourself aerobically *or* anaerobically, which is why your body doesn't seem to make progress even if you do get tired during your workouts.

Fitness routines aren't rocket science, but they are a science. We don't want you to have to worry about any equations, so we did the work for you. Only this time, you won't wonder why you're getting results—you'll just wonder why it took so long to figure out a better approach.

REJECT THIS THOUGHT:
Supplements are complete bullshit.

---

* I just want it on record that Bornstein wrote that particular pun. My narcissism goes only so far. —JR

DON'T HATE THE CARDIO, HATE THE FITNESS GAME

We just told you that cardio isn't ideal for fat loss, which is why our program will take a more efficient approach to giving you the body you want while still allowing you to eat the foods you love most. But that doesn't mean traditional cardio is bad.

As much as we're frustrated by the overblown claims regarding slow cardio, we're just as pissed at the experts who say there's no place for that type of physical activity. These people posit that you can get the same benefits from weight training, dieting, swinging kettlebells, surfing, horse training, or having sex that you can from long-distance cardio. In other words, they're just as deranged as the cardio lovers mentioned above.

The fact of the matter is, there are benefits from running that you can't get from anything else—such as getting better at running. While all the other types of exercises listed are good for fat loss, if properly used and programmed correctly, longer, slower bouts of cardio can be used not only to help with fat loss but also to support recovery and blood flow to enhance the efficacy of the program as a whole. And it's a hell of a lot better than sitting on your ass.

Short bursts of high-intensity exercise are fantastic. But they have limitations because *intensity* is a relative term that differs on an individual basis. Most trainers work with people who are in an untrained state. How much sense do you think it makes to take these people who haven't worked out and tell them to sprint as fast as they fucking can for thirty seconds—which, by the way, is longer than many Olympic sprinting races last?

In other words, while high-intensity interval prescriptions are great in theory, in practice they need to be applied strategically and cautiously. This extends beyond sprinting to include biking, stair climbing, hill running, and interval weight training.

Right off the bat, we see that moderate-intensity cardio has some benefit, if at the very least as a tool to progress to more intense exercise and modalities. Going beyond that, we still believe that there is a lot of merit to keeping your body in motion for long periods of time. Even if sprinting causes no injuries, your body will get good at running for short periods of time but not for long periods of time. And these limitations can show up in other areas of your life. You won't be able to play a game of flag football without getting hurt. Want to run a charity 5K? You can only run the first 300 yards.

That's why a balanced approach is the best approach, which is exactly what you'll find in the workout programs starting in chapter 8.

We love alcohol ads, and it's not because we love alcohol. Whether it's Dos Equis promoting the Most Interesting Man in the World or Patrón portraying a life with you as a baller, alcohol brands understand how to sell image without negative backlash. Those ads facilitate a world of partying and fun, which are elements of a lifestyle that people desire. No one actually thinks that drinking Dos Equis will make you savvy or that ordering Patrón will guarantee that beautiful women will throw themselves at you. You're smart enough to know that's not the case; and yet you don't criticize the alcohol as a crap product because of an unrealistic, sensational sell.

The ads you see for alcohol—or almost any other consumer good—are no different than what you'll find on supplement ads. The models in supplement ads don't look the way they do because they took that particular product. You know this, and yet the marketing techniques used to sell supplements oftentimes end up with the products condemned as useless.

Like anyone else who's been involved with the fitness and nutrition business for a decade or more, we've developed sort of a love/hate relationship with supplements—and supplement companies.

On the one hand, we love supplements (when they do what they claim), and without the convenience of protein drinks, meal replacements, vitamins, and the occasional protein bar, many people would struggle to reach their goals given all the demands and barriers that exist in busy lives. On the other hand, a lot of supplements are just flat-out crap. They're filled with only half of what the label says, and who knows what the other half is. And of course, many supplement companies have shady marketing tactics like Photoshopped before and after pics and other underhanded BS—and we're just not into that.

Having said all that, if chosen wisely and used correctly, supplements can make your program even more productive and can accelerate your progress. The companies we recommend are certified GMP (Good Manufacturing Practices). With this rating, you know for certain that you're getting exactly what the label says—and nothing it doesn't—every single time. You can find a GMP stamp on the front of the packaging or on the back next to the nutrition information. One thing is certain: it won't be hard to miss. Manufacturers that have a GMP certification want to boast about it because it's very valuable.

WHAT'S GMP AND WHY IS IT SO IMPORTANT?

There's a reason we make such a big deal about GMP, although most people who buy supplements have never heard of it. All supplements play in a very ambiguous space where they can't be strictly regulated by the FDA, which is why you find so many supplements making crazy claims and occasionally getting in big trouble because of ingredients that weren't on the label.

That is, unless they are GMP certified. This is how you know not only that a product is good but also that it's pure. By definition, certified GMP supplements take the hard road to getting the thumbs-up on quality.

"These regulations, which have the force of law, require that manufacturers, processors, and packagers of drugs, medical devices, some food, and blood take proactive steps to ensure that their products are safe, pure, and effective. GMP regulations require a quality approach to manufacturing, enabling companies to minimize or eliminate instances of contamination, mix-ups, and errors. This in turn, protects the consumer from purchasing a product which is not effective or even dangerous."

—FDA

That's one of the biggest reasons we love these supplements and why having a GMP stamp on the products you use should help you sleep better at night.

Also, you won't find products from these companies in mass-market supplement stores—and with good reason: products found in those stores need to come in at a certain price point to hit the right demand mark. This means, effectively, that brands must water down their products to fit the mold and make profit through those stores. By avoiding those stores and selling *directly* to customers, though, they're able to keep costs down, and as a result, use the proper doses needed for the products to get you results, whether for muscle, strength, power, fat loss, energy, or vitality.

Your decision to take or skip supplements will not make or break your body—but they can be a difference maker. Although there are very few supplements that will actually help your body work more efficiently and provide that extra edge, they're the only ones you need.

The Alpha Guide to Supplements

■ *THE ALPHA MALE STACK*

Protein Powder

Why You Need It

Protein is one of the foundational blocks of any good diet. It's what helps you build muscle. It's what helps you lose fat. And it's what allows you to stay lean, keep full, and avoid binging on foods that you'd be wise to avoid other than on cheat days. Now, there is nothing magical about protein powders other than the fact that most people don't eat enough protein in their diet. And these drinks, which now taste much better than they did ten years ago, can be used as a delicious way to provide your body with all the protein it needs with a dessert-like flavor. You just need to make sure that you find high-quality proteins. Research shows that the best approach is taking a blended protein powder that digests at different speeds so you make the most of the supplement.

Our Recommendations (www.engineeringthealpha.com/protein)

- BioTrust Low Carb
- Trutein
- Jay Robb

Greens Drink

Why You Need It

Everyone should be taking a multivitamin. You probably know this by now. But the rules of multivitamins have changed. The problem with multivitamins is that your body can't take advantage of all the vitamins and minerals listed on the label, and it doesn't absorb most of the nutrients. That's why a greens supplement is a better route. All the nutrients are derived from whole fruits and vegetables, making it a more natural route for your body. It's a superfood that will boost your overall health, improve your immune system, protect your digestive system, and help you fight off a variety of diseases. And those are claims that no multivitamin can make.

Our Recommendations (www.engineeringthealpha.com/greens)

- Athletic Greens
- Greens+
- VegeGreens

Fish Oil

Why You Need It

Sometimes you don't need to rant and rave about why a product is so important to take. That's the case with fish oil. Research has shown the following benefits:

- Less inflammation
- Improved recovery from exercise
- Less body fat
- More muscle
- Better-looking skin
- Higher sex drive
- Better brain functioning
- Less disease

Let's cut the chitchat. Just do yourself a favor and take fish oil.

Our Recommendations (www.engineeringthealpha.com/omega3)

- Athletic Greens Omega3
- Nordic Naturals

Vitamin D

Why You Need It

Men don't get enough sunlight. And this has nothing to do with having a great tan. The sun provides your body with vitamin D, and recent research indicates that more than 40 percent of men are deficient in vitamin D, according to the journal *Nutrition*. This wouldn't be an issue if vitamin D wasn't so essential to your health. Low levels have been linked to cancer, cardiovascular disease, heart attacks, and depression.

And research from Canada now shows that people with higher levels of vitamin D also have lower levels of body fat. The connection isn't coincidence. Vitamin D helps you feel fuller because, according to Australian researchers, it helps you release more leptin—an important hormone you'll learn about in chapter 5. And it also helps you store less fat by decreasing parathyroid hormone, which makes you hold on to lard. Best of all, vitamin D literally burns more fat by reducing production of the stress hormone cortisol, which you'll also learn more about in chapter 5.

Our Recommendations (www.engineeringthealpha.com/vitaminD)

- Athletic Greens D3
- Nature Made D3

You can't target specific areas of your muscles.

Judging the past by the standard of the present, Arnold Schwarzenegger and his crew were certified broscientists, in the sense that nothing they did was scientifically validated and they just used observation. You see this all the time; the big guy at the gym has some "proven" thoughts on what will work best for muscle growth. There isn't any science behind it, just years of experience, testing, and experimentation.

While this can be helpful, the best approach is one that combines real-life experience with science that can explain the results. And while bodybuilding pseudoscience has persevered for years, without science, it makes it harder to prove the cause of results. We finally have some answers to explain why some of the methods actually work.

In a somewhat ironic scenario, science is now telling us that the broscientists (bodybuilders) were right—more interestingly, that even when they were wrong, they weren't necessarily far off the mark.

Let's look at one of the hallmarks of traditional bodybuilding workouts: selective hypertrophy. As early as the 1950s, bodybuilders have been staunch in the notion that varying exercises and body positions on exercises can target distinct areas of individual muscles, preferentially recruiting specific fibers during the movements. For close to twenty years, though, you've been told not to do that. And the only reason was that there wasn't scientific research to back up the results.

One of the most difficult aspects of the fitness industry is that the experts are divided. One group focuses on what works, and the other on what can scientifically prove what's effective. Ideally, you are able to marry the two. But oftentimes that takes time. All scientific research needs to be funded. And earning that funding is a long, difficult process. Not to mention, a lot of the cool stuff that you would do in the gym would never get funded because most research companies just don't care about muscle building and fat loss the way the average guy does.

This led to a divide in that being pro-research meant accepting an anti-bodybuilding slant on fitness techniques. For example, because it hadn't been exhaustively concluded that incline pressing worked the clavicular head of your pecs, the very idea was considered foolish; study-dependent coaches maintained that muscle fibers run the entire length from origin to insertion and are activated by single nerves, and as a result they said it is not possible to preferentially recruit specific areas. Of course, that is possible, as every bodybuilder in history has known.

Now, research is clearly showing that some coaches and scientists owe those bodybuilders an apology. In a review paper written in 2000, Dr. Jose Antonio began to dispel the misconceptions and demonstrated clearly that you *could* target areas of specific muscles.

In the time since that paper was published, much more research has emerged to substantiate Antonio's position, and this is finally working its way into the public eye of the fitness industry, thanks in no small part to a group of fantastic coaches who are doing their best to get the information out there.

One such coach is Bret Contreras,* who regularly contributes to the largest bodybuilding magazines in the world. In a recent presentation, Bret said:

> It is now readily apparent in the literature that all muscle groups . . . contain functional subdivisions which are preferentially activated during different movements. . . . recent research has shown that altering body position such as foot placement . . . can target different areas of muscles. Bodybuilders were right all along; it just took research some time to catch up to their wisdom.

Contreras's assertion makes clear the fact that it's time to revisit a lot of what we consider myths and, with a critical but open mind, evaluate if we were not wrong in dismissing them for lack of evidence. After all, as much as we love science and research, we also love results. And you shouldn't question the validity of what works just because it hasn't been tested.

REJECT THIS THOUGHT:
You need to eat before you train.

One of the most common questions we hear is, what should I eat before I train? To that we have a somewhat roundabout answer.

The real question should be, do I need to eat before I train?

If you're like most people (and that includes us), eating before a workout is more of a burden than a convenience. Yes, we love food, but we also hate waiting two hours for our food to digest. And then when we train—especially with high-intensity or fat-loss protocols, we really hate feeling so sick to our stomach that we have to revisit our pre-workout meal.

So why do people stress about eating so much? In this case, we can blame the research. There's a whole bunch of science that shows eating before a workout creates an environment that helps you build muscle and burn fat.

And that's true. But what is considered "before a workout" is a much wider time range than you might think.

In the simplest sense, your digestive process is very complicated. When you eat, the food does not go directly to your muscles or your gut. It takes time—a lot of time, in fact. So if you eat many hours before you train, there's actually still plenty of fuel to help you train

---

* Bret, consider this your official shout-out.

and for you to build muscle. And there are many factors that influence your rate of digestion, such as your activity level, age, stress, and even the size of your body.

Research published in the *International Journal of Sport Nutrition and Exercise Metabolism* looked at the rate of digestion of protein. The study revealed that the type of protein you eat digests at a rate of anywhere between 1 gram per hour and 10 grams per hour. (So you know, whey protein digests the fastest, whereas egg protein lasted the longest.)

Do the math, and if you have a meal consisting of 50 grams of protein, that meal could last in your system for anywhere between five and fifty hours. That's a big range, but it gives you an idea of how your pre-workout meal can happen many hours before you train.

Now, that's not to say that eating before you train is bad or won't help. It will. But the amount won't be so significant that you'll notice any changes in your body. Trust us— neither of us eats right before we train and it's clearly not hurting us. In fact, if you believe the research on fasting before training, *not eating* before a workout helps you recover faster from your workouts and makes your muscles more efficient. You see, when you eat before you train, you teach your body to require a certain amount of protein and carbohydrates to lift more weight or run harder. When you learn to train with less energy (by not eating as close to your workout), your body adapts and learns to train harder with less fuel. Your body will adapt and pull from other stores for energy (such as fat), and then utilize your carbohydrate and protein stores more efficiently. The result: more muscle and less fat. The dream scenario that you want and we've promised.

If you're still worried about not eating before training, understand this: when you fast before you train, your levels of hydration and sleep patterns play a significant role in your performance. In fact, poor sleep or not drinking enough can have a bigger negative impact on your ability to train hard than not having a protein shake before your workout.

If you want to eat, go for it. And if you're concerned about potentially losing a little bit of muscle, then follow our lead and take BCAAs (Branched-Chain Amino Acids, the building blocks of protein). They are not necessary, but they get the job done. And what's more, researchers from Syracuse University found that simply adding amino acids before you train boosts muscle gain and fat loss. The study looked at two common meals before your workout: one with carbs (think: a sports drink) and one that combined BCAAs and carbs. After the pre-workout meal, the subjects then hit the weight room with a focus on heavy resistance training. Think: max weights that scream testosterone.

After the training, several important factors were examined, including muscle gain, fat loss, and metabolism. While both groups saw benefits from what they ate before a workout, it was the BCAA group that saw a bigger improvement in every measure. But maybe most impressively, those who had BCAAs before training saw a greater increase in their metabolism up to forty-eight hours *after* they finished training. While research has known for a while that weight training improves metabolism after a good workout, the surprising benefit was that those who took BCAAs (like BCAA Matrix) pre-workout had an increased metabolism the following day—above and beyond the normal surge experienced from weight training.

WHAT SHOULD I EAT PRE-WORKOUT?

We understand that some of you will still want to eat before you train, and that's fine. Just keep in mind that if you eat something immediately before you train, it won't really help your workout. The food will still be in your stomach and not digested. That's not to say there's no benefit; psychologically you might just feel better, which is part of the equation. If you eat, aim for at least an hour before you exercise. Here are three go-to meals for those who want a little fuel before hitting the iron.

The Quick and Easy: Greek yogurt and a handful of almonds

Simple Chef: Three scrambled eggs, ½ cup oatmeal, and ½ cup berries

The Power Shake: Frozen banana, chocolate protein powder, handful of almonds, 1 tablespoon cacao powder, 4 ice cubes; all blended

WHAT ABOUT PROTEIN BARS?

Do you like Snickers bars? Awesome. We do too. But Snickers bars are about as healthy as most protein bars. Don't be deceived by nutrition labels, which can hide a lot of dirty ingredients. The truth is, most protein bars are loaded with as much—if not more— sugar than your favorite candy bar. The only difference is that the health bars include more protein, which certainly is a good thing. But even then, the protein in the bars is oftentimes inflated. Ingredients like gelatin are included in the protein total. And while technically gelatin can count as protein, it's not the type of protein that builds muscle.

Solution: the Alpha Bar.

We teamed with YouBar, which creates custom-made, all-natural protein bars. The Alpha Bar is the type of protein bar you want: not too high in calories but still packed with all the good proteins, carbs, and fats for hormonal optimization. There are two variations: the Alpha Bar (for any situation) and the Alpha Workout (for after you train).

If you want something similar (and not made by us because you're afraid we might have dipped our fingers in the batter during the production process), we highly recommend Quest Bars. They are some of the highest-quality bars—without the added crap—that you'll find on the market. To find the Alpha Bar, visit www.engineering thealpha.com/alphabar.

REJECT THIS THOUGHT:
Crunches give you abs.

There is nothing inherently wrong with crunches. Let's just start with that. You can do crunches and they'll work your abs. Within the last five years, crunches—the perpetual king of abdominal exercises—have been criticized for everything from being a waste of time to causing back pain and even playing a role in the collapse of the economy. (Okay, so maybe the last one isn't true.)

In a world where the backup quarterback is always the most popular player on the team, planks stepped in as the savior for all your abs' needs. They promised no more back pain, 100 percent activation of your six-pack muscles, and anyone could do them. They were new, different, and difficult. Only one problem: crunches work your abs. It's a fucking fact. Research published in the *Journal of Strength and Conditioning Research* found that crunches create 64 percent activation of your rectus abdominis—the six-pack muscle. And when you add weight, that percentage increases.

Whether crunches target your abs is not the issue—it's whether they make your abs visible. You've probably heard that everyone has abs, but it's hard to believe when people will crunch and crunch and crunch and still don't have abs. But the problem isn't exercise selection. They could be planking all day, doing hanging leg raises, or med ball slamming their way to China and they wouldn't be able to tell a visual difference from one exercise to another. That's not to say that these exercises don't work your abs in different ways—they do. But seeing your six-pack does not depend on if you selected the "right" abs exercises.

Seeing your abs is a matter of lowering your body fat. Drop your body fat to around 10 percent and you'll see your abs. Lose even more fat and they'll really pop. You've probably heard that we all have a six-pack and that it's just covered by fat. That is true. Just as we all have biceps and pectorals. But you have to train those muscles, build and grow them, and strip away the fat to reveal your handiwork.

The Alpha program—which consists of four specific training phases—eliminates all the smoke and mirrors. Our workout isn't filled with exercises that you feel but can't see. We address the six-pack solution by combining exercises that are proven to burn fat. And this isn't just what you find in the lab. We're talking about the thousands of clients we've worked with. These are science-tested and real-life-approved strategies that offer results you can't deny. Whether it's metabolic complexes that leave you more exhausted than sprints, heavy strength work that you'll feel in your abs more than a thousand crunches, or innovative exercises you've probably never tried before (hello, hack squat), you'll be wondering why we've kept all of this a secret for so long. But we haven't. This is just the first time you've had the opportunity to work with us—and similarly, it'll be the first time you'll be able to say good-bye to your fat and hello to your abs.

SHIT YOU NEED TO KNOW

You don't need to be the smartest guy in the room to make an impact, but you never want to be the dumbest guy either. Here are some things you need to know. And tell your friends while you're at it. These facts dispel some of the worst myths that, simply put, need to die. We won't bother addressing these mistruths in detail because they've been discussed so often. But we realize many people reading this might be new to fitness, and that isn't a crime. So here are the facts that will steer you away from BS advice and keep you sounding smart and acting smarter:

- Fat doesn't make you fat. It's necessary for hormonal balance.
- Heavy weights don't make you bulky. Don't fear them; they are your friend.
- Yoga is not just for girls. Yeah, we said it.
- The bench press is not the king of all chest exercises (try the push-up).
- There are muscles in your legs. Work them—especially your hamstrings and glutes.
- Muscle does not weigh more than fat. But fat does take up a lot more space than muscle.

PART 2
REBIRTH

"WHAT YOU REALLY FEAR IS INSIDE YOURSELF. YOU
FEAR YOUR OWN POWER. YOU FEAR YOUR ANGER,
THE DRIVE TO DO GREAT OR TERRIBLE THINGS."
—HENRI DUCARD, *BATMAN BEGINS*

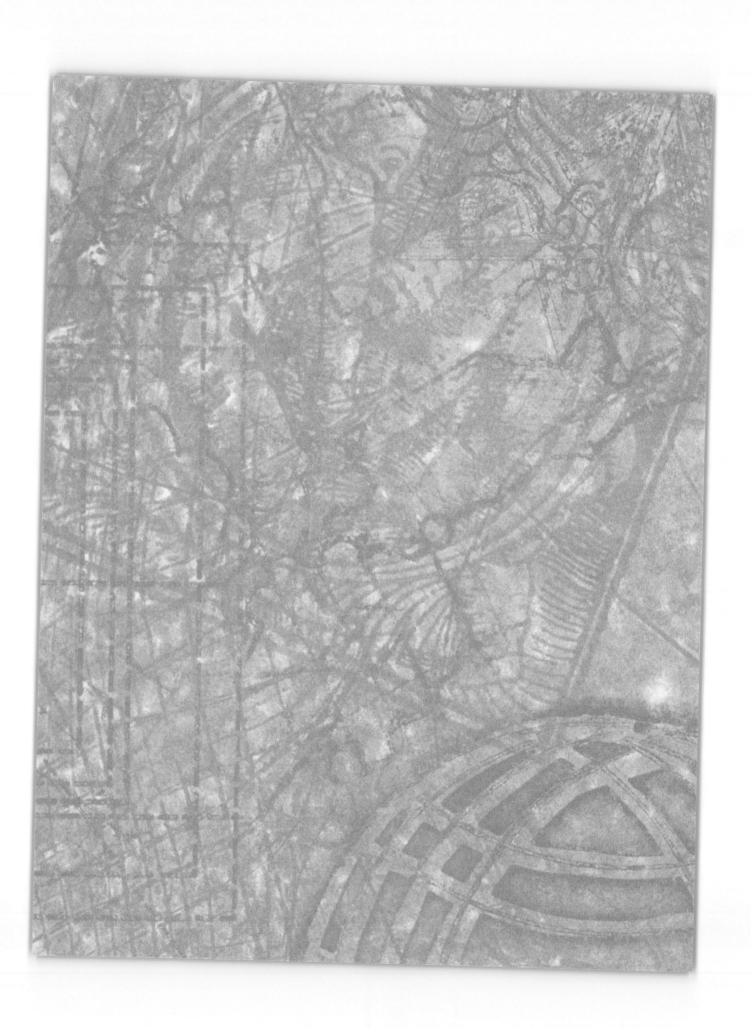

CHAPTER 4

The Call to Adventure

HOW THIRTY WHITE POLO SHIRTS
CHANGED ROMAN'S LIFE

*"Some people can't believe in themselves until
someone else believes in them first."*

—*GOOD WILL HUNTING*

ice to meet you, Roman," the lady said over the phone. "I'm in a bit of a rush, so I hope you can help. I'm going to need thirty white polo shirts, in different sizes. Mostly medium and large, with some small and extra large. Probably just one or two extra small. I'll be there in fifteen minutes."

It was a very strange request, on a strange day, in a strange time in my life. It was May of 2001. I was nineteen years old, and in the summers between semesters, I worked at my old high school job. The worst job I've ever had. I was working—of all places—at the Gap. I was the jean-folding drone rocking the big smile at the register. Not exactly my preferred job description, but it was my reality. I had been home from school for nearly two weeks and was unfortunately slated to be home for quite a long time. In fact, I had transferred to a local school for what my transcript says were "personal reasons."*

While my grades didn't take a huge dip, my motivation and confidence did. I had no idea what I wanted to do and no desire to pay $40,000 to figure it out. It seemed logical, but two weeks into Gap slavery, I was regretting my decision. Local schooling meant corporate servitude, and low-level corporate servitude, at that. My prospects looked grim. I

---

* That's a nice way of saying I was incredibly depressed and had trouble focusing on everything.

was twenty-five pounds overweight, pissed off at the world, and desperate to change something, anything, *everything* in my life.

And if dealing with anger, depression, confusion, a gut, and a healthy dose of teenage angst wasn't enough, now I had this lady sending me down to the fucking basement of the fucking Gap to search for thirty white fucking polo shirts.

It took me twelve minutes to find them all, even though we only had twenty-seven. Emerging from the cool, dark depths of the stock room laden with my perfectly folded cargo, I found the lady from the phone waiting for me at the counter.

A short Italian woman with an infectious laugh, Marie—as I would later learn was her name—made it nearly impossible for me to remain grumpy. After all, anyone who reminds me of my own mother can put a smile on my face.

I rang up the shirts, and I asked the obvious question: "Soooo, um, what does one need thirty—er, twenty-seven—white polo shirts for?"

Turns out, her husband was opening up a gym. And after further questioning, I found out that it was merely five minutes away from my house.

None of this would have seemed bizarre except for the fact that earlier that day, I'd mentioned to my best friend that we should join a gym and get in shape. With a swipe of her American Express and a friendly wave good-bye, she was gone and I was left with my thoughts.

Two days later I walked into that gym, and in many respects I have never walked out.

DISCOVERING YOUR MENTOR

Marie's husband was a man named Alvin. Good-looking and exceptionally well built, he was the first man over forty I had ever met who lifted weights seriously. Alvin shook my hand and showed me around the gym. As we passed the bench press, I mentioned that I held the school record from my high school football days. He gestured to the bench, "Show me what you got."

Perhaps that was a sales tactic of his. And perhaps my acquiescence was some innate need to impress him. I pumped out 225 for three reps while Alvin spotted me for the first time—but certainly not the last. He patted me on the shoulder, took care of my paperwork, and I was now a member of his gym. But more importantly, he was now a member of my life.

Three weeks later, Alvin offered me a job, and all of a sudden I was working at the gym in one of those crisp white polo shirts, cleaning equipment and selling memberships. It wasn't the most glamorous work, but it was better than the fucking Gap.

That very day, Alvin would become my Obi-Wan, my Mr. Miyagi. He was my first mentor. He gave me books, taught me lessons, and paid for my first personal training certification. He introduced me to magazines I would later go on to write for. He encouraged me and pushed me.

I worked at that gym for many years, first part-time between semesters and then, when I finished school, as a full-time trainer. I learned more there than at any other place in my life. I learned about training and how to work with clients. I learned sales and how to deal with people professionally. I discovered how to manage a staff, and started my first business there. Finally, when I was ready, I eventually left to start a new venture that led to this point.

THE CALL

It wasn't until years later, when I was writing a blog on Campbell, that I realized my life had changed because of thirty white polo shirts. That phone call, however strange, set into motion a series of events that pulled me from my depression, changed my body, and shaped my life.

That phone call introduced me to a place and an industry where I would find a home. And it helped me create a skill set that I could use to help others for years to come. In some ways, this book is because of that phone call.

Are you ready for your call?

In every person's life, there are calls. Some are literal—like mine—and others are figurative. Perhaps it's not quite as obvious as Princess Leia's plea for the aid of a Jedi Master, but it doesn't matter. Your job is to be aware that such calls exist. And when they arrive, you must rise up to the challenge and listen to the opportunity. I heard the Call to Adventure in that very moment in the Gap, and responding to it changed my life in every way possible.

Now it's time for you to hear yours—and to accept the challenge. We're here to make sure that you won't miss out on the greatest journey of your life—and that you make the decision that can change everything.

MAKE MORE MONEY, HAVE MORE SEX, AND BE FUCKING AWESOME

The Call to Adventure is a nebulous thing. It can be loud. It can be soft. It can be obvious—but it is usually not. And because it is not usually obvious, it can be missed.

The call is different for everyone because it's dependent on reaching a breaking point and coming to a realization that you want to make a change. In terms of improving your body, it can be something subtle, an external motivator, like seeing Arnold materialize in *The Terminator*. For others, it might be the internal desire to get on a field and play a sport. For a good many of our clients, it was the moment when they looked at a picture of themselves on vacation and realized "how bad it had gotten." And for others, the call comes in the form of a slap in the face (hopefully verbal) from their doctor.

All these signs have one thing in common: there's no turning back after that moment.

ENGINEERING THE ALPHA

SUBJECT: *Andy Edwards*

THE ORDINARY WORLD

I remember the day vividly; there I was looking in the mirror on a warm sunny March morning wondering who the fat guy was staring back at me. The sad thing was: I thought I was eating okay and exercising regularly, and yet if you looked at me you wouldn't have believed it. I was thirty-six, hated what I saw in the mirror, and knew it was only going to become worse. This was my life. It seemed good and comfortable, but deep down inside I knew better.

Like most people who don't have the balls to leave their comfort zone, I continued exactly the same diet and magazine workouts. When results didn't come, I just told myself I needed more time. Depressingly, nothing had changed, including my waistline. And this pissed me off.

ACCEPTING THE CALL

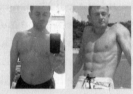

It was at this point that I realized something must change drastically. I had to check my ego at the door and realize I didn't know what I needed to do. Or to be more precise; I knew what to do, but not how to do it. I needed help. Once I had realized this, I only had one question: Who?

Enter Roman. I immediately felt connected to his non-preachy, witty, and personable style. Within a few short months the transformation was insane. My body fat had dropped from about 18 percent to 8 percent and has remained below 11 percent ever since. I had a huge moment of pride when a gym trainer asked what the hell I was doing, as he couldn't get the same results with his clients.

ALPHA STATUS

Although "The gym is a metaphor for life" is cliché, it's extremely accurate and poignant. My physical transformation didn't just affect my body; it improved all areas of my life. Initially, looking better was great for my personal vanity. I also noticed a significant increase in my self-confidence, and that is the true value I took from this change.

Once I started to feel better about myself, literally everything improved, from my personal relationships, my career, attitude to life, and my general worldview. I started to feel like the Alpha version of myself. I was now living intentionally and with a purpose, not just spinning my wheels. I had drive, ambition, and focus. I had become everything I ever wanted, but never knew existed.

In *The Writer's Journey*,* Christopher Vogler says, "The Call to Adventure establishes the stakes of the game." For people who have heard the call, that seems obvious.

The sad truth, however, is that the majority of people live their entire life without ever seeing the sign or hearing the call. And as a result, they never realize what's at stake.

We recognize that for many people, this book may serve as the Call to Adventure. And in this way, we fulfill the role of the herald; it's a responsibility we don't take lightly. If by now we have not made it abundantly clear, let us explain in plain English what you stand to gain by accepting the call.

See Your Abs

Let's just get this out of the way first: having abs is awesome. Sure, it's a superficial goal. It doesn't make you stronger or better or smarter. But abs are the hallmark of a good body. And having them gives you unparalleled confidence. After working with clients for more than ten years, we've learned that most people don't actually consider themselves in great shape until they have abs. So we're going to help you get them.

You might think that your body isn't made for abs. That's not true. Or you might have heard that seeing your six-pack emphasizes form over function. That makes no sense. We believe that every muscle has a function. Fuck the haters who say that having abs is useless. It doesn't matter if the form of your abs is to help fight diabetes (more on that soon) or if the function is helping you get laid. Either way, having abs has served a function in your life that is important to *you*. Which is exactly why seeing your abs is part of the plan and why you'll be happier when you can. End of story.

Build Muscle

Many people typically over- or underreact to the idea of building muscle. We're not here to sell you on the idea of looking like a bodybuilder or an athlete. Your goals are up to you, and we respect that. Whether you want to be jacked or just lean like a surfer, you need to build muscle. Here's why: muscle is your armor. It protects you from disease, it protects you from obesity, and it protects you from insecurities that undercut your confidence and can strangle success.

And that is why having a muscular body is important. By balancing your hormones, all these problems can be avoided and your specific goals for how you want to look can be achieved. If you have more testosterone, it's easier to have a hard body. And by increasing GH, you potentiate your testosterone growth for better results. Add in improved insulin sensitivity, and you'll find that as you add muscle, you also can burn more fat and look leaner.

* Absolutely one of the best books on Campbell you will find, anywhere. Subtitled *Mythic Structure for Writers*, Vogler's work has been an invaluable resource throughout Roman's career, including the writing of this book.

Remember, whether you want to gain two pounds or twenty doesn't matter. What does is appreciating that muscle is directly tied to your health and your goal appearance. Everything is relative to what you want, so if you're not looking to get huge, remember that all of this advice still applies to you. And if you are looking to pack on some serious mass, this program will also do the trick—and you might want to repeat it a few times for optimal results.

If you want to find out how, flip to part 3 and you'll see the workouts from this program that make this happen. But we still suggest patience because understanding what's at stake will allow you to take full advantage of our program. Remember, this isn't just about blindly following some awesome workouts and a diet plan. It's about becoming the Alpha, learning why and how to become better, and being able to pay it forward to help others. And that's impossible if you don't see the entire picture.

Have More Sexy Time

In most books, the typical start to this section would say something along the lines of, "If we have to convince you to have more sex, then you're not much of a man (har har har)."

But this isn't your typical book.

You can have as much or as little sex as you want. The real problem is that you don't *desire* sex as much as you used to or as much as you should. Low sex drive is a very common problem, and just as disturbing is the fact that it's infecting men at a younger and younger age.

Low sex drive is primarily the result of low testosterone, but it's also impacted by other hormonal factors. Fortunately, all your sex drive problems can be turned around with a concentrated approach that increases your testosterone.

Lest we lead you to believe that we are just a couple of oversexed meatheads who spent a few too many years as the go-to resource for the information in *Men's Health*, here's what you need to realize: sex is very important. And not just because it's awesome and feels great. Your sex drive is linked to self-worth and self-confidence. It's a psychological and sociological fact that virility and masculinity are tied together, and those factors are closely linked to your confidence. And as we've already established, your confidence is deeply tied to your success. You'll learn in chapter 5 just how much these foundational elements are the catalyst for creating and living an unreal life.

Wanting sex is not just important as an individual. Sure, if you're a single guy and you don't want sex, you should be worried. Your sex drive is what will make it possible to meet the one (or, hell, many partners) that you're looking for in your life. But when you're in a relationship, sex is important to your overall well-being and the strength of your relationship too.

A lack of intimacy can lead to a metric fuck-ton* of problems that—please believe us—you do *not* want in your life.

---

* A unit of measurement roughly equal to 2.18 metric shit-tons.

ALPHAS WANT SEX

Not just frequent sex, but *good* sex. Alphas want sex to be meaningful to them in a number of ways. Whether you quantify that by performance or connecting with your partner, great sex is something that Alphas are great at. Put somewhat less delicately, Alphas are fucking *great* at fucking.

Before you get the wrong idea: we're not telling you that you need to fuck a lot of girls. That's not for us to decide; remember, part of being an Alpha is setting your own expectations for your ideal.

We don't really care whether you want to have a new partner every week or the same one for life. Your sex life is *your* sex life. What we care about is helping you make sure that it's a *good* sex life, because no matter how you slice it, sex is an essential part of life and something you can't ignore. And we think that this is a large issue that needs to be addressed.

So how do you solve it? First you need to acknowledge the problem. Stop living in denial and start taking action. Then, realize that you don't need to visit your doctor or take shots or use creams. You can fix everything with some dietary tweaks and lifestyle changes that will optimize your hormones and boost your sex drive to where it should be.

Increase Confidence

As you learned in the Alpha Traits, there is a marked difference between confidence and cockiness, and it's important to realize that optimizing your hormones sets you up to be more confident. Whether you become cocky is up to you.

Confidence is an honest appraisal of what can and can't be achieved. Confident people don't have a sense of entitlement or an ego that pushes people away. Instead, they have a mind-set that creates opportunities and inspires other people to become better.

Case in point, in business, confident people don't think that they can run a business without training for it. Instead, they know when they deserve a promotion because they've worked hard and can point to their contributions with full conviction and resolution.

In social situations, confident people know they can talk to others—whether it's a complete stranger at a party or the most beautiful woman at the bar. That doesn't mean you walk around thinking you're the greatest thing in the world and should be banging models.* Instead, confidence is about thinking you're interesting and using that opinion to hold a conversation and engage with others. Confidence is a trait that opens up a world that you want.

---

* A generally disappointing experience, anyway. —JR.

Optimizing your hormones is the gateway that can make this confidence a reality—rather than a dream.

Sleep Better

We probably don't need to tell you that lack of sleep can screw up your life. You know that it makes it harder to concentrate and work, but you may not know that it also messes with your body on levels that directly impact your ability to lose fat. When your sleep quality is poor, your metabolic rate decreases, making it easier for you to pack on pounds faster than you can say, "McDonald's." A bad night of rest also limits your ability to recover from your workouts, meaning it becomes harder to become stronger and build more muscle.

But the biggest problem is tied to your hormonal production. You see, there is an implied catch-22 when it comes to sleep quality and hormones—particularly cortisol. If you have high levels of cortisol, you have trouble sleeping. And when you don't get enough sleep, your cortisol levels rise. Cortisol increases during times of stress, and one way stress creates itself is insomnia.

You don't have to be a sleep expert to see how it's a perfect storm to ruining your rest on a nightly basis. It's a vicious cycle that can be hard to break, and for many people it is the underlying reason for why they don't have the body they want.

But all hope is not lost. If you can take the steps needed to balance your hormones, you can offset even the most ejaculatory production of cortisol. (Yeah, we said *ejaculatory*.) What's more, we're going to teach you some simple strategies that you thought were bad—such as late-night eating—that will not only help you sleep better and longer but will also make you leaner.

Need more convincing that sleep is essential? Researchers at the University of Warwick and the University of Naples Medical Schools found that people who sleep fewer than six hours per night have a shorter life expectancy. If living longer isn't a good enough reason to focus on your sleep, then we don't know what is.

Improve Your Skin

Listen, it's fine to want to be a pretty boy. We'll admit that we have an array of skin products that we use to look good. But that's not the first step to improving your skin; instead that's the final line of defense. If you have a bad diet, you produce toxins that ruin your appearance.

Sure, you could take products, but that will only address the symptoms of bad skin. Having great skin starts from the inside; it's a by-product of increasing GH, optimizing insulin sensitivity, and reducing your cortisol. These changes will not only reduce pimples; they will also improve elasticity, which helps you look younger as you age.

Now is not the time to get sensitive, but we're about to point the finger at you.

If you're like most guys who struggle with their weight or simply have difficulty looking the way you want, odds are, you have an eating problem. And it's not necessarily that you eat the wrong foods—it's that you eat too much. And why do you eat too much? Well, it's because you're always too damn hungry. Whether you wake up needing food, scavenge for snacks at work, or come home famished, your stomach seems to be in perpetual starvation mode.

And that's because it is.

Recent research has found out one of the main reasons why you're always hungry, and it has nothing to do with what you're eating. The problem is how you're sleeping. Research published in the *Journal of Clinical Endocrinology and Metabolism* found that a lack of sleep impacts your brain in a way that pushes you toward a "see food" diet, which explains why you always want to eat.

Just how bad is it? Only one night of insufficient sleep (fewer than six hours) triggers an area in your brain that is involved with your need to eat. Unfortunately, this is just the tip of the iceberg. A lack of sleep also increases ghrelin, a hormone that increases appetite, while decreasing leptin, the hormone that keeps you feeling full. This is what allows you to keep on eating . . . and eating . . . and eating . . . even as you put more energy (food) into your body.

It's mind control, and you have no solution other than to get more rest. Or you'll be forced into a world where you desire more food when you don't need it. Focus on getting at least six hours of sleep. Make it a priority as part of your program, and you'll quickly find that your hunger pangs will subside after each meal.

As you might know, many people consider GH to be the fountain of youth. But the benefits aren't limited to less fat and more muscle; it literally makes you look younger. So if you improve your hormonal environment to produce even more GH, then you can slow the visual effects of the aging process. This is the reason most men look younger than women as they age—they naturally produce more GH.

And the benefits don't just directly influence how you look. As we mentioned before, proper hormone balance facilitates better sleep quality. And when you sleep better, your skin also improves. And that's what we call a win-win situation.

Fight Diabetes, Cancer, and Heart Disease

As you're sitting reading this book, you might be increasing your risk of diabetes. No need to read this book standing, but it is a good reminder that seemingly everything we do these days increases our risk of disease or shortens our life.

Which is why you need to do everything you can to combat a lifestyle that is literally killing you. Before you head to the doctor and file for your hypochondriac's license, how about you try something a little cheaper and research-supported to build armor against the world's most dangerous diseases?

You see, researchers at Harvard found that combining weight training and cardio in the right doses—which we followed for the programs in this book—can reduce your risk of type 2 diabetes by more than 59 percent. The reason is insulin sensitivity—which we've already mentioned as one of the most important hormonal factors you need to control. Insulin sensitivity reduces insulin resistance. And reduced insulin resistance has been strongly linked to avoiding disease. We're not talking about the common cold. Insulin resistance may be the key to preventing prostate and pancreatic cancers—two of the most common forms in men—and warding off diabetes and heart disease.

Anyone can claim that exercise fights off disease or that they are combining cardio and weights in the right doses. But we've gone a step farther to create a synergistic environment that is scientifically proven to keep you healthy. That's because we'll also be combining variations of intermittent fasting. Don't let that word scare you. This simple eating strategy has been shown to help prevent diabetes, according to research published in the *American Journal of Cardiology*.

As we discussed in chapter 1, we'll help your body spend more time in an autophagic state, where your body is constantly healing and cleaning out the garbage. Autophagy is a by-product of intermittent fasting, which protects your cells from the oxidative stress that is typically the cause of cancer, diabetes, and heart disease.

Not to mention, the latest research from Harvard has identified a new hormone called irisin. This hormone promotes insulin sensitivity, which speeds up your metabolism. But more importantly, irisin transforms white fat into brown fat. Even though you might not even realize that your body has two forms of fat, you do. The white stuff gives you love handles and the brown gives you a six-pack. Simple, right?

But here's the best part about brown fat—you can control its presence. A study published in the journal *Nature* found that contracting your muscles—like you do in any exercise from squats to sprints—produces a substance called PGC1. Do you care what PGC1 is? Probably not—unless you're trying to impress a hot scientist—but PGC1 is the secret to stripping away your gut. PGC1 produces a protein called FNDC, which then breaks down into several components, including irisin. And irisin is exactly what will turn your white fat into brown fat, transforming you from a man with a belly to a man with flat abs and bigger biceps.

Brown fat isn't just about looking good naked, although we fully endorse that motivation. When scientists were able to create more irisin in rats, it prevented diabetes even when the scientists were *purposely* trying to create the disease, according to a study performed at Harvard Medical School and published in the journal *Nature*.

The effect was so powerful that the men and women in lab coats are trying to find a way to bottle irisin and turn it into a weight-loss medication, but there's no timetable on how long that might take. In the meantime, the easiest way to produce more irisin is to increase activity and hit the weights hard and heavy. That's what the eggheads at Harvard have concluded—that your muscle cells communicate to your body fat via irisin. Strength training can generate more irisin, and it will literally transform your bad fat (white) into the good stuff (brown).

This is where we come in to play. We've read the studies and talked with the researchers, and we designed this program that will prime your hormones to make you healthier and help you fight disease—while simultaneously making sure we're taking advantage of their abilities to aid in weight loss and have you look fucking amazing. Our program is the result of more than ten years of testing these strategies on clients. And for the last four years, we've fine-tuned the hormonal-based approach and seen consistent results with hundreds of clients. Now it's your turn.

Boost Intelligence

Some of the smartest and most successful people in the world also happen to be the fittest. Look at Richard Branson, Mark Cuban, and Tim Ferriss as three prominent examples. Some might chalk this up to pure coincidence. We're not part of that crowd.

You might have heard that your brain is a muscle. Although doing bicep curls won't make your brain any bigger, it will keep your brain active—which is like steroids for your mind.

While many people simply assume that slowing brain function is a natural part of aging, it's actually something that starts in your thirties. And one of the best ways to prevent your brain from hitting snooze is to stay active. Canadian scientists found that physical activity and burning calories are directly linked to boosting brain activity and fighting off Alzheimer's. The reason is simple: exercise promotes blood flow. You know this because when you do curls you feel the pump—that's just more blood going to your biceps. But that blood flow isn't limited to the muscles you're working; it occurs throughout your body, which includes your brain. The blood flow in your brain promotes activity, and that activity keeps you sharp and smart, rather than dull and aloof.

That's how exercise and your hormones directly influence your mind. But the indirect benefits are just as important. That's because as you become heavier, the extra fat on your waist does not just slow down how quickly you move—it also slows down how quickly your brain works. That's the message from the American Academy of Neurology. When analyzing more than six thousand people over the age of fifty, the researchers found that those with more fat experienced 22 percent more cognitive decline than those who were normal weight. Although the study didn't investigate why this occurred, prior research sheds some light onto how a poor diet is not only bad for your stomach but also terrible for your mind. Your weakened brain might also be affected by your avoidance of healthy foods. Scientists at the University of Oregon found that better brain size and function are directly related to diets high in antioxidants, vitamin B, and omega-3 fatty acids.

Does this mean that fat people are stupid? Of course not. Our brains are capable of some incredible feats, and slowing down cognitive processing does not mean you lose the ability to function or even work at a high level. Some of the most brilliant minds are not people you'd see inside the pages of your favorite fitness mags. But remember that our approach is all about optimization and living up to your full potential. Do you want to take on life with one hand tied behind your back? We sure as hell don't. Life can be difficult enough, so we want every advantage we can get, which is why we share this information.

All of this is to say your diet and exercise program goes far beyond your looks and your general health. It literally controls how well your mind works—everything from mental acuity to the rate and intensity of your emotional fluctuations. Now, that may sound like something you'd read in *Cosmo*, but it's some serious shit. We will not only show you how to make sure you never fall victim to the deleterious effects of fat controlling your mind, but we'll also make sure that the natural diseases that occur with aging are less likely to take hold of your life. After all, researchers from the National Institute on Aging, in Bethesda, Maryland, discovered that intermittent fasting (yep, there it is again) protects your brain from cognitive decline, mental weakness, and diseases such as Alzheimer's and Parkinson's. And we're not talking massive changes—strategically dropping about 500 calories just two days a week can improve your brain health and keep you on top of your game.

Beat Depression

Remember how we just told you that your hormones would make you smarter? Well, the same hormone that influences your intelligence—BDNF—also could prevent you from feeling depressed. Now, before you start with some unsubstantiated claims that guys don't get depressed, understand that the national rate of depression has been trending upward for men, and NIH researchers estimate that between 7 and 10 percent of men are currently depressed. Think about that—that means about 1 out of every 10 of your buddies is depressed. And that's just clinical depression. Feelings of loneliness, sadness, or extreme frustration could easily be affecting many more people.

BDNF is your body's natural antidepressant. In fact, when you take antidepressants, those drugs signal BDNF to increase in your hippocampus, which is the part of your brain where depression occurs.

So how are we going to increase BDNF? Once again, through the power of intermittent fasting. Strategically timing your eating patterns—in a way that fits your schedule—will cleanse your brain so it signals feel-good hormones to keep your mind feeling good in spite of any stressors in your life.

Make More Money

You've probably heard that people who are taller make more money. What the hell does this have to do with anything? Well, for one, neither one of us is tall. So if you were feeling a little down, we were hoping this would level the playing field. But more importantly, while you certainly can't control your height, there are several other factors that can be improved by hormonal optimization and will help you fill your bank account as you build your biceps. And these factors are ones that you *can* control.

Whether you like it or not, the working world is influenced by appearance. Research shows that people who are perceived as more attractive make more money. And while beauty is certainly in the eye of the beholder, certain traits and characteristics are universally associated with looking good. It's why scientists have also found that people who are overweight make less money and are more likely to be perceived as dumb. Is this a fair judgment? Of course not. In fact, we think it's a little crazy.

But we tell you this because this is your frustrating reality: the aesthetic image you exude and the perception it creates are influencing your ability to earn higher-paying jobs and workplace advances. In fact, a study by Professor Vasilios Kosteas at Cleveland State University, published in the *Journal of Labor Research,* found that people who exercise and are rated as "in shape" make on average 10 percent more salary per year than people who aren't.

What's more, the researchers took their study a step farther and determined that the more time you spend in the gym, the more money you earn. Based on their calculations, working out three times per week increases your earning potential by 20 percent.

The reasons are numerous. Exercise improves brain health, confidence, energy, and even your mood—all of which are positive attributes in the workplace and for those deemed fit for upper management positions.

Translation: your health is literally your wealth.

But muscles that you can see through your suit aren't necessary to become an executive. Simply optimizing your hormones and becoming the Alpha create the confidence you need to climb the corporate ladder. Confident people make better decisions. And in the office, the more good decisions you make, the more people will respect you and the more your superiors will notice your work. In the end, success isn't always about the smartest and most competent person rising to the top; we know plenty of broke, frustrated Ph.D.s.

If you look at our society's entertainment, bosses in the movies are usually overly confident but highly incompetent. That's Hollywood's commentary on the reality of the working world, the best example being Michael Scott from *The Office*. Confident people rise to the top.

Sure, money won't buy happiness. But confidence will drive your success, which will build happiness and ultimately leave you a richer person in every aspect of your life.

Reduce Stress

While money can't fix everything, it does solve the problem of not having money. Not having money causes stress. That's a simple fact of life, and it happens to be the leading cause of stress in individuals and in interpersonal relationships. Money is the leading cause of marital problems, leading to more divorces than any other issue. And when you consider that the divorce rate is greater than 50 percent, it's not hard to see how sorting out your finances is essential to your relationship and your health.

We've already explained how we're going to help with the money situation, and there are more details to come. For now, you must realize that your finances are an indirect stressor. We want to eliminate those, but we also want to attack your stress in a direct way. Stress is caused by a psychological awareness of a lack of control, which literally causes a physiological reaction that makes you feel awful.

You should never feel that bad. That's why we've designed a program that puts you back in control. We want you to feel like you can shift your world in a real way. By creating this new reality where you can effect change, you will successfully remove one of the biggest causes of stress from your life.

That all starts with a diet and workout approach that is so powerful that you have no choice but to feel better. If this sounds too good to be true, we understand. But this is legitimate science. Even if you've never worked out before, you've probably heard about endorphins. These feel-good hormones are produced by biochemical reactions that occur when you exercise. They can help offset bad hormones, like cortisol. We'll talk more about cortisol in chapter 5, but if you've stayed up late at night watching TV, you've probably already heard about cortisol. It's the pitch made in every single infomercial for a fat-loss product. Stop cortisol, and you stop fat gain. That's partially true, but those infomercials use twisted science and crappy supplements that really don't fix the problem.

Put simply, if you're stressed, you produce more cortisol, which makes you fatter, more irritable, and in need of about five espressos to start your day. If that wasn't bad enough, the presence of cortisol increases the production of more cortisol and causes more stress.

It's easy to see why we blame cortisol for so many problems, but there are simple solutions that are much more effective than pills.

Even if you've been crushed by cortisol for years, adding in certain exercise and diet strategies can reduce the impact of cortisol. Strategies like lactic acid training and intermittent fasting (see part 3) also produce GH, which further reduces cortisol. This cocktail will offset all the problems caused by cortisol and in particular will remove your belly fat. And if you've ever been stressed by belly fat, well that's just one less thing that you'll have to worry about.

OPEN YOUR EYES

Unlike many people who miss the Call to Adventure because they never see it—you no longer have that excuse. We have portrayed this as directly as possible in an attempt to help you do what you might think is impossible. The only way we could make this more obvious is if turning this page opened a holographic image of a princess asking for help. Or perhaps a small Italian lady asking for thirty white polo shirts.

CHAPTER 5

Discovering the Answers

EVERYTHING YOU NEED TO KNOW ABOUT HORMONES

LUKE SKYWALKER: *I'm looking for someone.*

MASTER YODA: *Looking? Found someone, you have, I would say, hm?*

NEW YORK CITY, 7:48 A.M.
JOHN ROMANIELLO'S APARTMENT

"**Well, *that's* not a fun way to wake up.**" Being called an idiot, that is. Which is what I was being called, more or less—and first thing in the morning, to boot.

Like every morning, I began checking my e-mail at 7:45. It was now 7:48 A.M., and I had sorted things into their correct folders, deleted the spam (no, I would not like a bigger penis, thankyouverymuch), and prepared to dive headfirst into the shit storm that is my inbox—until the very first e-mail stopped me in my tracks.

It was from one of my clients who had a rather simple message to share: I didn't know what the fuck I was doing.

Well, to be fair, he didn't say that *exactly*; it was implied fairly strongly, however, at least in the sense that incredulity and disbelief were evident in every line of the e-mail.

It was from Colin, a forty-nine-year-old powerlifter who'd decided for the first time in his life that he wanted to get lean. He signed up for my coaching program, and within twelve hours and six minutes of receiving his instructions—according to my sent mail log—Colin had sent a three-page e-mail telling me exactly what was wrong with everything I had designed.

Of course, he didn't specifically say, "Roman, you're wrong." Nothing so direct. Instead, he questioned everything I had laid out for his new workout program.

Colin wasn't aggressive, but he was defensive of his ideas, his understanding of the training world, and what he "knew to be true." My ideas ran counter to all that, and his perception—and, in a sense, his *ego*—was going to be difficult to reconcile.

Like anyone else, I am prone to experiencing the whims of ego, and so my first instinct was to be offended and indignant that anyone would question my work. That instinct exists in every person and in every profession. Again, it's ego. It's based on a feeling of being right—and believing you're right.

Like Colin, I felt challenged, felt like my understanding of the world had been challenged—and I felt the urge to push back. That urge was quickly sublimated.

Instead, I took a deep breath and put myself in Colin's shoes. I read through his e-mail again and quickly realized that he wasn't challenging *me* as much as he was declaring the way my program confronted his view of the world. And, in fairness, the program was radically different.

Colin was a competitive powerlifter, a guy who routinely benched 350 for 3 reps and deadlifted more than 450 pounds for 3 reps. He'd been training for years—more years than I had, certainly—more years than I had been alive, in fact. And everything he had achieved was based on his training methods and his thoughts on his approach.

My program was not based on those same principles, not dependent on what Colin "knew" to be true. In order to accept my programming as effective, Colin was going to have to accept the fact that what he had done in the past wouldn't necessarily work for his new goals. Colin had to accept the fact that there are different methods for different goals.

Accepting my program required Colin to resolve the dissonance inherent in his confronted worldview—that was going to be a challenge for him, and that was going to be his first step. And it was *my* challenge to help him accomplish that.

But before either of us could take that step, Colin first had to accept that I knew something he didn't—that someone twenty years his junior was privy to secrets he was not.

In order for *anything* else to happen, Colin had to accept my role in his quest: his guide, his friend, and his teacher. Just as Luke realized in that swamp on Dagobah, Colin had to realize—as you must—that Jedi Masters come in all shapes and sizes.

ENTER THE MENTOR

Within the context of the monomyth, the first real transition—the first step in moving out of the Ordinary World and into the Special World—is known as Crossing the First Threshold, which is stage four in the journey, for those keeping score at home.

At this point the hero (you) has been shown that there is more to life than what he's experienced. He's come to an understanding that although he may not live in the Special World, it *exists*—and that realization fills him with fear and longing in equal measure.

The hero is made aware that there's a world outside his job—or his farm or his hometown, or whatever other incarnation of familiarity he is bound to—that there's success outside his cubicle, that there's a body he can't (yet) see in the mirror.

Unfortunately, mere *awareness* isn't enough to pull the hero from the Ordinary World into the Special one. Crossing the First Threshold is often the hardest part of the journey, but of course it *must* be crossed in order for the story to advance—you must take the hardest step, the first step, in order to move forward in your development.

In many cases, the idea of moving past the familiar and into the unknown is too great and leads to Refusal of the Call.

At that point, the hero requires something—or *someone*—to help him get over the proverbial hump. It is no surprise that stage four often overlaps with another extremely important event: Meeting with the Mentor.

Work	Hero	Mentor
The Sword in the Stone	Arthur Pendragon	Merlin
Lord of the Rings	Frodo Baggins	Gandalf
The Hobbit	Bilbo Baggins	Gandalf
Star Wars: A New Hope	Luke Skywalker	Obi-Wan Kenobi
Harry Potter	Harry Potter	Professor Albus Dumbledore
The Karate Kid	Daniel LaRusso	Mr. Miyagi
Hook	Peter Banning / Peter Pan	Tinker Bell
The Lion King	Simba	Rafiki
The Monster Squad	Sean	Scary German Guy
Dracula	Jonathan Harker	Abraham Van Helsing
The X-Men	Wolverine/Cyclops	Professor Charles Xavier
Any Given Sunday	Willie Beamen	Coach Tony D'Amato
Major League	Wild Thing Ricky Vaughn	Jake Taylor
Rocky	Rocky Balboa	Mickey Goldmill
James Bond	James Bond	Q
Cinderella	Cinderella	Fairy Godmother
Men in Black	Agent J	Agent K
Myths of Hercules	Hercules	Chiron the Centaur
Clash of the Titans (1981)	Perseus	Ammon
Jerry Maguire	Jerry Maguire	Dicky Fox
Hitch	Albert Brennaman	Hitch

It should come as no surprise that mentors play a role in creating a better life. Almost every successful person has a mentor, and the mentor archetype—or wise man— appears with the hero in nearly every story you've ever heard, from antiquity to pop culture;* in fact, it's so familiar that it's sometimes easy to overlook just how ubiquitous it is. Just to drive home how important it is for a hero to have a mentor to guide him on his quest, we've compiled a list of examples from some of the most popular books and movies of our time (see chart on previous page).

In the above table, we touched on the first *Star Wars* film, but the relationship actually appears in nearly every episode. It changes a bit from film to film, but it's there. Here's a breakdown, arranged in order of the story's chronology:

Episode	Hero/Student	Mentor
The Phantom Menace	Obi-Wan Kenobi	Qui-Gonn Jinn
Attack of the Clones	Anakin Skywalker	Obi-Wan Kenobi
Revenge of the Sith	Anakin Skywalker	Darth Sidious
A New Hope	Luke Skywalker	Obi-Wan Kenobi
The Empire Strikes Back	Luke Skywalker	Master Yoda

In fact, the only episode that doesn't prominently feature the hero/mentor relationship is *Return of the Jedi*. The reason for this is that George Lucas is a bit of a Campbell geek and recognizes the importance of the monomyth storytelling—and at the point that *Jedi* occurs, Luke is already a developed hero.

No matter, Campbell—and apparently, most screenwriters—agree that mentors are hugely important, so whether it's Mickey or Merlin or Mr. Miyagi, this character is omnipresent. When it comes to Crossing the First Threshold, the mentor's encouragement is often needed to help bolster the hero's confidence, allow him to push through the internal resistance, and pass into the Special World.

This was the situation facing Colin. And it's probably what's preventing you from breaking down the barriers in your own life too.

You picked up this book for a reason. You have a very clear idea that what you're doing isn't working. People want change, and they look for it. But when a new reality doesn't immediately resonate, it's met with resistance. When something is too different from what they were doing, it can make the idea of evolution too unrealistic.

The only way to resolve that is to not think about the method or the process. The only way that you can resolve this issue is to believe it. And the only way to believe it is to stop thinking about what you're doing—and to start focusing on *who* you're trusting.

---

* The very word *mentor* comes to us from Homer's *The Odyssey*, in which the goddess Athena disguised herself as an old wise man named Mentor, who would aid Odysseus and Telemachus with sage advice.

Anyone can be a teacher, but very few can guide you toward success that you can see, understand, and replicate. Transparency is key, which is why we waited so long to create this book. We've seen enough mentors fail that we understand our social responsibility to do the research and guide you effectively. And now, that's exactly what we're here to do; to be your mentors and make sure that you see all the hurdles in your way, navigate around them, and provide solutions to your specific problems.

Ultimately, trusting your guide gets you over the hump, and finding a guide you can trust is the key. You don't need to believe the method at first. What you need to believe is that your mentor knows more than you do and that he has your best interests at heart. If you can come to that point, then you don't have to understand the process. You don't need to "get" the Force. You don't need to comprehend the physiological methodology of the insulin reset, how hormones work, and how your metabolism can be rewired. All of that can be taught. What can't be taught is overcoming mental hurdles. That can only be resolved with trust.

If you trust us, then let us take your hand and lead you.

We've earned the trust of all our other clients, Colin in particular. We had to justify the training, go through all of his concerns, overcome his objections, and let him know that we understood. And because we had demonstrated success with other people who had achieved goals similar to his own, he was able to establish trust. That allowed him to take the step, cross the threshold, and be willing to try the new methods even if they seemed outlandish or different.

To this day, Colin is the prototypical success story and a representation of a man who is living his best life.

ENGINEERING THE ALPHA

SUBJECT: *Colin Wilson*

THE ORDINARY WORLD

I have been lifting weights close to thirty years. Everything I learned was through trial and error in the gym. I was starting to feel my age (forty-nine) and the pain of lifting heavy every day. I wanted to take a break to let my body heal and to start taking better care of myself. One training goal I was never able to attain on my own was to get below 10 percent body fat and be totally ripped.

ACCEPTING THE CALL

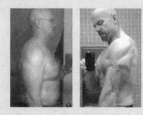

I knew I was going to need help with this, so I contacted John Romaniello. He is serious about his business and quite frankly he looks awesome, meaning he walks the walk and talks the talk. When I got the first month of training it was nothing like I was used to doing. There was nothing I would have even considered "lifting." I freaked a little bit; okay, I freaked a lot. How could a 280-pound guy be seen doing a goblet squat with a 30-pound dumbbell?

I have found that the training in this program requires a lot more mental discipline than I was used to putting in. Training for fat loss and to optimize your hormones is about pushing yourself through rep after rep, timing your rest periods, forcing your body to take on new challenges, and realizing that this program will change your body. Being able to do the hard when other people can't or won't is what it is all about.

ALPHA STATUS

I had complete strangers in the gym who watched me go through this journey come up to me and tell me how great I looked. One of the workers in the gym was astonished that I was able to accomplish so much in such a short time. I hit my goal of 9.5 percent body fat right at Christmas 2011, just six months after starting with John. I feel so much better now than I ever have. I never realized how much carrying the extra weight was affecting my life and health. I jump right out of bed in the morning and nothing cracks or hurts anymore. My numbers (blood pressure, cholesterol, O_2) are all those of a man twenty years younger. It has been over a year since I reached my goal, and I have been slowly adding more muscle to my frame while maintaining a very lean appearance. I have incorporated everything John taught me and have been able to change the way I eat and train.

WHY MEN SHOULD CARE ABOUT HORMONES

The signs of losing fat and gaining muscle manifest themselves on the outside, but how well or how quickly you do either of those is very much determined on the inside.

By understanding how your hormones affect you and learning how to address them through application of our methods, you will create change from the inside out.

Alphas consider the problem from all angles to find solutions.

We've already mentioned several hormones through this book, but now we're going to show you specifically why fixing your hormones will help you attain the life you want. But before we can do that, it's important that you understand the most important hormones in your body, what they do, and how they're already holding back your mental, physical, social, and emotional health.

■ *TESTOSTERONE*

We're not going to beat around the bush with this one: testosterone is what makes you a man. It's what allows you to build muscle and melt fat. It's what makes you attractive to women, what powers your sex drive, and what helps you recover from workouts. It's part of your genetics, and it's a driving force in your health, your wealth, your energy, and your life span. If it weren't for the existence of testosterone, we wouldn't be writing this book.

But we are writing this book because there's a serious problem. In the past twenty years, the average level of testosterone has dropped anywhere from 20 to 30 percent. And for that very reason, men have become fatter, less sexual, and less satisfied—with how they look, how they feel, and how they fuck. That's not an opinion; it's scientific fact.

And therein lies the problem with most approaches to health—they don't focus on testosterone. You can do all the reps and sets in the world, but if you're not producing enough testosterone, you won't add muscle to your body. It's the reason why women's bodies don't naturally bulk up. They don't produce testosterone like men do, and therefore their bodies look different. And as you'll see, your abilities to maintain and build muscle are essential to helping your body function better and creating the type of life you want.

Do not misunderstand us. Testosterone is not about becoming big and bulky like a body-builder. (Although it will help if that's your goal.) This is more about taking control of the characteristics that enable you to become the Alpha. Did you know that low testosterone levels can kill your sperm? Or that decreases in testosterone have been linked to decreases in brain activity and memory function? And men with higher testosterone have lower incidence of heart disease, spend less money on health care, and live significantly longer—we're talking potentially more than a decade longer.

Your testosterone levels peak in your twenties, but then they instantly begin dropping once you hit your thirties. The good news is you don't need to spend money to boost your T levels. Most doctors are overly quick to prescribe hormone replacement therapy and fill your body with exogenous hormones. But it's been shown that small changes—such as sleeping more—can be all it takes to increase testosterone as much as 50 percent. And that's just one simple change.

The primary goal will be eliminating your beer belly. The more fat you carry, the more aromatase you produce, which is an enzyme that converts your testosterone (the good stuff) into the female hormone estrogen. This is what will make you look softer, have softer erections, and even make you softer emotionally. And we know you don't want that. By cutting down on your fat, you'll have the greatest impact on ensuring that you continue to produce more testosterone and stay young as long as possible. After all, Australian researchers found that testosterone levels don't have to drop as you get older. In fact, they can stay high up into your sixties if you exercise the right way, eat the right foods, avoid smoking, and limit how much fat is on your body.

You'll find plenty of tips to increase testosterone in this book, but here's your cheat sheet to higher T.

- Lift heavy weights.
- Do intervals.
- Practice sprints and work your lower body.
- Supplement with Vitamin D (at least 300 IU/day).
- Don't smoke.
- Supplement with zinc.
- Sleep more than six hours per night.
- Eat more protein.
- Do squats and deadlifts.
- Use shorter rest periods in the gym.
- Take fish oil.
- Don't overtrain (just follow our program).
- Include fat from animals and dairy in your diet.
- Eat eggs.

■ *GROWTH HORMONE*

If testosterone is the Batman of masculinity, then you could say GH is your Robin. This powerful yet understated hormone is oftentimes considered the fountain of youth, as doctors and antiaging clinics prescribe it readily to help combat old age. GH and testosterone work best together, meaning that each is very potent individually, but when present together, the impact is decidedly more prominent and beneficial.

GH has been shown to have the greatest physical impact on burning fat and increasing longevity. But what's even more useful is what GH does to help your body function more efficiently and effectively.

When you have more GH circulating in your system, you're able to make better use of protein and build more muscle. You're also able to improve the quality of your sleep and speed healing and recovery. Like the name would imply, GH improves the growth of your cells—it helps grow muscle mass, strengthen your bones, reduce the pressure on your liver, and maybe most understated, protect your immune system. Increasing your GH is one of the best ways to fight off disease and stay healthy.

You'll learn many ways to improve your GH, the most impactful mechanism being the new style of eating called intermittent fasting that we'll teach you in part 3. In the meantime, here are some easy ways to boost your GH:

- *Sleep more.*
- *Fast during the morning.*
- *Improve sleep quality.*
- *Lift heavier weights.*
- *Supplement with BCAAs.*
- *Eat big before bed.*
- *Perform sprints (10–30 seconds are best).*
- *Do high-intensity metabolic resistance training (30–40 minutes max).*
- *Don't eat fat before a workout.*
- *Don't eat too many calories before exercise.*

■ *LEPTIN*

We've all seen a friend drop twenty pounds with ease and then have trouble losing the next five, right? Perhaps it's even happened to you. It's frustrating to experience, and like most weight-loss phenomena, its roots are linked to your hormones; specifically, a hormone called leptin.

Named for the Greek word *leptos*, meaning "thin," leptin is produced in your fat cells—which means that the more fat you have, the higher your baseline levels of leptin will be. Here's why this is important: one of the master hormones, leptin influences the production and secretion of other hormones that regulate metabolism, such as thyroid hormones T3 and T4. When leptin levels are high, your production of T3 and T4 will also be relatively high, allowing you to burn fat faster; when leptin levels drop, these other hormones go too.

The fact that leptin is produced in fat cells is an important reason why it's easier to drop weight when you have more excess weight to lose. However, leptin levels also share a direct relationship with caloric intake—when you eat fewer calories, your leptin levels drop considerably. This, in turn, lowers your other fat-burning hormones, bringing your fat loss to a crawl.

For this reason, leptin is often called the anti-starvation hormone—your body is slowing your metabolism to keep you alive when food is scarce. This means that leptin decreases your hunger. That's great for survival, but it creates a pretty clear fat-loss catch-22: you need to eat less to burn fat, but eating less compromises your body's ability to produce leptin. And the less leptin you produce, the hungrier you become and the more likely you are to eat more than you need.

All of this means that if you want to keep making progress, you need to keep leptin levels elevated while you're in a caloric deficit—and we'll show you how to do exactly that in chapter 7. For now, keep these leptin-boosting tactics in mind:

- Fast at least sixteen hours a day.
- Include strategic cheat meals (maximum of one day per week).
- Perform resistance training.
- Perform long-distance cardiovascular training.
- Avoid anabolic steroids (yes, they are illegal; and yes, they decrease leptin).
- Eat a high-protein diet.
- Don't eat too much fructose.
- Don't drop your calories too low on a diet (at most, drop 500–600 calories per week).

■ GHRELIN

Of all the hormones, ghrelin is the most fun to say because it sounds like gremlin. And, like gremlins, it's an annoying little bugger. Known as the hunger hormone, ghrelin is produced in your hypothalamus (located in your brain), kidneys, and pituitary gland, but most of it is synthesized in and released by the stomach, and it is released in a pulsatile manner *throughout the night, peaking when you wake. No matter where it's produced, it always has the same effect: snack attack.*

You see, ghrelin both induces hunger and is also secreted by it. Your stomach produces ghrelin when it's feeling empty. Whenever you start producing ghrelin, you'll feel hungry— and anytime you get hungry, ghrelin is secreted. Now, here's the important thing: your ghrelin secretion schedule largely follows your eating schedule, because ghrelin is what we might call a trainable hormone—the more often you eat, the more often you'll produce ghrelin.

This is one of the many reasons why the multiple-meal hypothesis—the one that states you need to eat five to six mini-meals per day—is flawed. This style of eating—from a hormonal standpoint and in light of the way our bodies are built—is designed to make you hungrier. This might be great if your goal is to gain weight. In that case, you want to be hungrier. But if losing weight and becoming leaner are your goals, training your body to eat less frequently, while still feeling full, is a more sustainable and enjoyable approach to eating without feeling frustrated or constantly hungry.

A better meal schedule will help you balance your ghrelin levels, and so will sleep. Research published in the American Journal of Human Biology *found a direct link between a lack of sleep, overeating, and obesity. Many people think the reason less sleep leads to more eating is because when you sleep less, you're awake longer; the more hours you're up, the more time you have to eat. The real reason is that a lack of sleep impacts hormone levels and brain functioning in a way that pushes you toward more foods—and in particular the crap you should avoid.*

It's a three-pronged attack designed to make you fat. When you don't sleep enough:

1. *Cortisol levels rise, which activates reward centers in your brain that make you crave food.*

2. *You produce more ghrelin and it's harder to decrease the levels, meaning you feel hungry all the freaking time.*

3. *The lack of sleep and higher levels of ghrelin appear to make you more likely to grab for dessert foods and fattening, sugary snacks.*

While cheat foods will have their place in our program, the goal is for you to eat them when you want—not because your brain creates a desire that you can't resist. But that's exactly what happens when you don't get enough sleep. When researchers from Columbia University used MRI testing on sleep-deprived participants, they found that the areas of the brain that desire junk food were more activated with less than six hours of sleep. So unless you want to be a mind-control experiment that is at the beck and call of every fast food commercial on television, your best protection is ensuring more rest.

Here's how to prevent high ghrelin:

- Ensure enough sleep.
- Avoid eating too much sugar.
- Don't eat too often.
- Eat more protein.
- Practice intermittent fasting.

■ ESTROGEN

You might know estrogen as the female sex hormone that is at least partially responsible for the development of breasts. You know, because men love breasts. Estrogen also regulates the menstrual cycle and the female biological love of chocolate. (Seriously.) All of those things are awesome—in women. But estrogen is also present in all men (yes, we need it), and it's an essential part of hormonal balance—in the right amounts. However, when men's estrogen levels are too high, they can wreak havoc on the male body, in ways that include the growth of man boobs, decreased libido, and depression.

Estrogen is one of the most interesting hormones because of its necessity combined with its potential downside. Estrogen is essential to your ability to produce sperm. Without it, those little guys just won't exist. But when you become too fat, the enzyme aromatase will convert your testosterone into estrogen, and that's when things start going bad.

In the next chapter, you'll learn the immediate strategies you can use to supercharge your testosterone, keep estrogen levels at bay, and keep your body as manly as possible. After you learn those easy-to-apply strategies, we'll jump immediately into all the eating details that will reshape your body and mind. These will include carbohydrate cycling, strategies to improve your digestive health, the supplements you need to keep testosterone up, the best protein sources, the right types of exercises, and even the types of alcoholic drinks you should be consuming—all of which will keep your estrogen at optimal levels.

For now, keep your estrogen low with these easy tips:

- Avoid soy.
- Limit stress.
- Stay happy (depression increases estrogen production).
- Don't eat too much bran or too many legumes.
- Watch out for toxins from plastics (translation: avoid eating out of plastic containers).

- *Eat pesticide-free or organic produce.*
- *Eat lots of broccoli and cauliflower.*
- *Limit alcohol.*
- *Eat red meat.*

■ *INSULIN*

"Insulin—that's the carb hormone, right?" Well, sort of. Insulin is about more than just carbs—it controls everything from how quickly you can lose fat and gain muscle to whether the food you eat gives you energy or makes you crash.

Produced in the pancreas, insulin is responsible for the uptake of nutrients into cells in your liver, muscles, and stored fat. For this reason, insulin is sometimes known as the gate-keeper hormone. When insulin is working efficiently, your cells are primed for nutrient storage. So if you utilize insulin at the right time, like immediately after a workout, you'll direct nutrients into your muscle cells. Even if you don't like exercise, controlling insulin is the key to looking good. That's because if you raise insulin levels at the wrong time, it'll be your lipid (fat) cells that uptake the nutrients, regardless of whether you're training like a champion or perfecting your couch-surfing skills.

Unfortunately, the timing of insulin mastery isn't as simple as some people would make it seem. That's because insulin doesn't occur in a vacuum. The goal is to make your body more insulin sensitive. When insulin sensitivity is high, you need less insulin to get the same effect. High insulin sensitivity is the easiest way to ensure that you'll gain muscle, not fat. You can increase your insulin sensitivity by avoiding foods that cause a high spike, such as sugar, and lifting weights to build more muscle. Your muscles are your best friends when it comes to burning the fuel you put into your body—especially carbs.

But most people have diets that are constantly spiking insulin levels in a way that confuses their bodies. And while many people exercise, they do so in a way that doesn't improve their insulin sensitivity, which, as you'll see, is the real secret to better fat loss and muscle gain. If your insulin levels are screwed up—which is a problem that plagues most people without their awareness—then even your post-workout carbs can be detrimental and dangerous.

The goal then becomes learning how to manage your insulin so you can take advantage of it at the right times. Chronically high insulin levels will result in something called insulin resistance. This means that your body uses insulin less efficiently, so you need to produce more in order to digest and utilize carbohydrates effectively. This is not good. You don't want more insulin pumping through your body. You only want insulin effectively shuttling the foods you eat in an advantageous way. So because you're producing more, it just means the foods you eat are more likely to be stored as fat.

When you are insulin resistant, your blood sugar levels stay higher for longer periods of time because the carbohydrates you eat (which turn into glucose in your body) are slowed down and don't make it to your muscle cells. This is literally how you become resistant. Your muscles are the engines, and the carbs are the fuel. If carbs become backed up in your transport system, then you become less efficient at storing your food the way your body wants (as muscle). When that happens, your fuel system becomes backed up with carbs, your arteries become clogged, and the carbs you eat are stored as fat because your body literally has no other choice.

It's a vicious cycle because insulin resistance shuts down your body's ability to burn fat. So if your muscles aren't receiving the carbs—because your body is resistant—then you produce more insulin and those carbs and sugars are stored as fat.

Even worse, it's not just that your body is getting fatter. It's also having trouble building muscle. Those same carbohydrates that are getting trapped in your bloodstream are also blocking your ability to transport proteins and amino acids to your muscles so that they can grow, recover, and help your entire body work the way it should. And because your muscle cells need sugar to grow (remember, carbs are fuel), your body feels that it needs to create sugar. How does it do that? (Wait for it . . . wait for it . . .) By breaking down muscle in order to provide your body the sugar it thinks it needs to function. Only problem? You have the sugar, but it's trapped. So you hold on to the sugar as your body eats away at your muscle.

Oh. Fuck. Not so hard to see why we become fat, right?

Inevitably, your body craves more and more carbohydrates as you become more insulin resistant. And it's not your fault. You're trying to feed the machine (your body), but the equipment isn't working right, so your body is literally plotting against you. And if you think having screwy insulin management only affects your physique, you'd be underestimating the power of the dark side . . . we mean insulin. It can cause problems with everything from your boners to your brain. Oh yeah, and you can die . . . of the beetus.*

Our entire goal in the diet and exercise portion of this book will be showing you how to manage and control insulin so it's your bitch. And by that we mean you won't have to worry about everything you eat turning into a ticking time bomb. Instead you'll be able to eat carbs, proteins, and fats, and your body will use them in a beneficial way.

---

* If you have no idea what we're talking about, do us a favor and Google "Wilford Brimley diabetes commercial." While diabetes is not funny, "the beetus" certainly is.

■ *CORTISOL*

If you've ever watched infomercials at two A.M., you've heard of cortisol. The so-called stress hormone is a bit of a double-edged sword, particularly with regard to its relationship with fat.

Produced in your adrenal glands, cortisol is primarily a catabolic agent. Although the word catabolism *is normally associated with muscle loss, it simply refers to the breakdown of substance for energy. This can certainly relate to muscle, as prolonged elevation of cortisol has been definitively shown to lead to proteolysis, or muscle breakdown; however, short periods of elevation have been shown to lead to lipolysis, or breakdown of fatty tissue. And if there's any type of breakdown we love, it's of fatty tissue.*

There's also evidence that links cortisol to the storage of abdominal fat. In other words, if you have high cortisol, you're likely to store most of your fat on your belly. All of this makes cortisol an interesting hormone when you consider that producing it can break down fat and help you get lean . . . or it can cause you to store fat in the worst area.

What makes cortisol even more complicated is that you want it to rise during activity. It is directly linked to your fight-or-flight mode, which means that when cortisol rises, you can use that stress to improve your performance. This is a great thing for your training, as you want more intensity. But if cortisol remains elevated for too long, it causes a rise in blood sugar, which makes you crave all sorts of unhealthy foods, according to researchers at the University of Southern California. What's more, it can make you insulin resistant. And as you already learned, insulin resistance is a badass motherfucker that you want no part of.

The question, then, is how do we ensure that it's used for increasing performance and not for ruining our bodies? Simple: you manipulate cortisol through diet and training. And we'll teach exactly how to do that starting in chapter 8.

THE TWO BIGGEST REASONS YOU DON'T HAVE THE BODY YOU WANT

We'll be blunt—if you're struggling to become the man you want to be, chances are your efforts are being sabotaged by two foundational problems: metabolic slowdown and program stagnation. Before you can even begin optimizing your hormones, you need to key in on these two areas.

Metabolic Slowdown

At their core, most programs aimed at fat loss are based on a single thing—what we call energy deficit. Simply, you need to burn more calories than you take in. It's this principle that allowed Kansas State professor Mark Haub to drop weight on his highly publicized Twinkie Diet. In fact, it's upon this principle that all diets theoretically function.

Theoretically.

For someone like Haub, who wants to drop from a soft 33 percent body fat to a soft 25 percent body fat while starving himself by subsisting on a few Twinkies a day, then sure, that principle works. As a matter of fact, it works for just about everyone who starts any diet at all, Twinkies or not—for a little while, at least.

But if getting lean were as simple as eating less and doing more, everyone would be walking around with a six-pack. The truth is that at some point, fat loss stops, and for most people, that point is sooner rather than later. After a few successful weeks of dieting, the scale stops moving.

After all, no matter how long you've been on a diet or how close you are to your goal, the real determinant of success is how balanced your hormones are. Hormones in check are the real secret to unlocking the "unrealistic" changes that separate the ordinary from the elite.

When you're in a calorie-reduced state for an extended period of time, your body eventually starts to rebel against you. This is because leptin drops dramatically. And just like that—*bam*—fat loss stops dead. This is what's often referred to as starvation mode.

Sadly, almost every man who has ever tried to exercise and diet has experienced the phenomenon. Had Haub (a professor of nutrition, by the way) stayed on his exceedingly brilliant nutrition plan of snack cakes and irony, he would have hit the unfortunate wall with a crash. But it's not limited to gimmick diets. Even people on regular diet programs—you know, like all the ones you've tried that have left you frustrated—reach a point where fat loss stops.

Once you get to a certain level of leanness, other hormones come into play. As mentioned, estrogen keeps men from developing their testosterone-fueled physique, instead resulting in man boobs. Insulin (or rather, resistance to it) keeps love handles right where they are:

attached to the waist—or even worse—causes metabolic syndrome and threatens to shorten life. And perhaps worst, stress-enhanced cortisol keeps your abs covered in flab—because it's cortisol that prevents all people from losing belly fat.

Ever known anyone who was just trying to lose the last few pounds? Of course you do. Well, those people are the victims of their hormones. And unless they do something about it, those last few pounds will be there forever—their adipose tissue will adapt, making it harder and harder to drop those pounds.

Something else to consider is that these things don't just affect the way you look; they affect everything else, starting with your health. Here's a brief list: insulin resistance is the first step to diabetes; high estrogen is a factor in a host of cancers; and belly fat resulting from cortisol has been linked with metabolic disorder, heart disease, and brain degradation. Oh, and if that wasn't bad enough, all three hormones can lead to erectile issues.

Not addressing these hormones isn't just keeping you fat; it also might kill you. But if you *reprogram* your hormones, you literally have the chance to upgrade the way you look, feel, and age.

Program Stagnation

On the reverse side of the coin, the guys trying to build muscle have it just as hard as those trying to lose fat. That's why the term *hard-gainer* exists—because for some people, gaining muscle seems to be the most difficult task in the world . . . when it should be the easiest.

The motto for gaining muscle should be easy: eat big, lift big, get big. But it's not. Once again, hormonal issues control the speed at which you gain muscle.

But the average guy at the gym doesn't know that. In fact, he doesn't know anything. He just does what seems to come naturally to him—what he's always done.

This guy starts out with the same program he used for high school football. He has no idea why he's not seeing results; he just knows he's not. So he steps it up and jumps onto a program from a magazine. He doesn't know why he picked that program; he just thought the exercise model looked good. Again, this guy knows nothing, so he doesn't know if it's a good program—he also doesn't know enough to match his diet to that program. So, again, no results.

Time for a new program, right? Hey, if it's broke, why fix it when you can just replace it?

This is a phenomenon known as program hopping—which is when clients move from program to program to program, often without finishing any. Even when they do finish a program, these hoppers don't really think about the overall structure of their training as a whole. They move to whichever program seems cool at the moment.

The problem with this is that even in the best-case scenario, even if one of the programs works for this guy, he's going to sabotage his results by either staying on it too long or moving on to something that doesn't make sense.

He has no idea about periodization, which models each workout you do so it's built on the one before it—your results stack on top of each other, and everything becomes successively more effective.

But our guy doesn't know that. He has no idea about periodization. He has no idea what he's doing isn't just ineffective . . . it's counterproductive.

How counterproductive?

Well, let's look at the worst-case scenario. Our guy has no idea about anything . . . so he has no idea that the program from his favorite muscle magazine might be intended for steroid users. He has no idea that with his natural hormonal levels, he can't hope to even recover from it, let alone gain muscle. He doesn't realize that instead of just being a waste of his time, this program will lead to overtraining, a phenomenon that will put him in a worse situation . . . because overtraining forces hormones like testosterone and GH to drop lower and others like cortisol to creep ever higher.

This combination can lead to even lower hormonal levels and a worse physique. But guys just keep doing it, because it's what they've always done.

In order to reverse the trend, men have to stop doing what they've always done. No more programs that only go for four weeks. No more generic nutrition advice. No more acting like the human body plays by certain rules—like you can't eat after 7 P.M.—that have no scientific basis. There are some rules, but there's also lots of freedom to find a sustainable plan that works for you, without having to follow a bunch of dogmatic rules that would make you miserable.

Most importantly, there's plenty of proof that an Adonis lives within every man and that any feelings of underachievement can be overturned once the hormonal switch has been flipped.

CHOOSE YOUR PILL

We realize that our program might sound like a stretch. Or you still might not understand the processes of metabolic slowdown or program stagnation. Maybe GH and testosterone still sound illegal. But they are two of the most natural hormones known to man. And we'll teach you all of this—and how to make your body work in ways that you've always wanted.

At this point, you need to make only one decision: believe that a better body and a better life are very realistic options and that there's a reason for *every* previous frustration and doubt that has stood in your way before.

If you've reached that point, then you're ready to leave your ordinary world, knock down the barriers, and progress to the type of life you've always wanted—and never thought you could have.

CHAPTER 6

An Unreal Life

HOW TO BE MORE AWESOME
AT BEING AWESOME

"After a certain age every man is responsible for his face."

—ALBERT CAMUS

hen we first started the process of pitching this book—combining the ten years of experience and findings into the one concise* document that you now hold in your hands—our book agent had one major question: How could we possibly promise guys an unreal life?

From day one, it was the primary rallying cry, the reason why we felt this book needed to be written. We knew that we had developed a program that could literally transform your body from a physical standpoint; but for us, that wasn't reason enough to write a book. There are tons of fitness books, and even more of the diet variety. And there are lots of great websites with information. Hell, you can visit either of our websites for some of that knowledge. And there are many others that have played a key role in our education. (See our acknowledgments if you want to know our preferred sources for fitness and nutrition information.)

But we wrote this book because our unique approach to training and diet had a synergistic effect with a far-reaching impact that went beyond looking fucking amazing in a mirror. We found that, as we changed bodies through hormone optimization, the domino effect reached into areas of life that we could have never assumed. Once was an aberration.

* LOL, "concise."

Twice was nothing too impressive, maybe even coincidence. But then the list grew to literally hundreds of success stories. And when we say success, we literally mean success.

Men had changed their lives. They had become more than who they had been before and beyond what they'd thought was possible.

Turns out, hormone optimization is the holy grail for living an unreal life. It sounds crazy, but read the rest of this chapter and then you can judge for yourself.

LIVING THE DREAM

We define an unreal life as having a level of success, confidence, and happiness in every aspect of your existence that means something to you. Our goal is to help you create a level of satisfaction so that you sit back and wonder, *how is this real?*

That's an unreal life—and that's what we're going to provide.

It means having the sex drive of your prime, a brilliant mind that works efficiently, and the body of a god.

Great. Now how does that actually happen? After all, if it were that easy, there'd be no reason for us to explain that it's not impossible.

There's a fundamental flaw in how we were taught to achieve things. Despite plenty of clichés that preach quality over quantity, our behaviors still drive us toward a mentality that focuses on doing more, achieving more. Want more money? Work harder. Want bigger muscles? Do more reps. Want to meet more women? Ask out more girls.

Fortunately, life doesn't have to work in a linear fashion. In fact, stepping back from this quantitative approach has endless benefits.

So what's the missing piece? The fact that you're not searching for a missing piece. If science has taught us anything (and trust us, despite the wealth of research in this book, we know that life is not experienced in a lab—but truths are supported there), it's that the most important relationship is cause and effect.

It's not: What do I have to do to reach my goal?

Instead it's: What's the catalyst that makes everything come together?

We're going to put an end to the typical cause-and-effect behaviors you see. Such as when you want better sex, you pursue more women. If you want a better body, you buy a gym pass. If you want to get smarter, you take a class.

Your frustrations are globally linked to a mind-set of *how* you approach your goals and desires. And in order to overcome those problems, we're going to provide the exact outline that will put things in motion. Think of it as a domino effect. It's not that you weren't knocking down dominos before; you were just hitting pieces that weren't the backbone of the entire system. Once you find the right trigger point—that's when things really get started.

So where does it all begin? The answer is sex.

SEX AND THE SELF

When it comes to being a man, sex is probably the most misunderstood subject, both internally and externally. Like it or not, men are Neanderthals. We mean that in the nicest possible way—but not the paleo way.* We intrinsically link the definition of our manhood to our sexual prowess, our ability to attract and sleep with women, and even the size of our penis. Men define their manhood by their manhood—and everything that stems from it.

The desire for sex can be a force that encourages and propels you to do great things, such as achieving a high level of success or power. But it can also be destructive. The drive to have women can derail you from your quest to become the Alpha by diverting attention away from your goals of improved sense of self and achieving your potential. More than anything else, women bring out the competitive, comparative nature that typifies the traditional perception of the Alpha that we want to rewrite.

This very battle is illustrated in the Hero's Journey. The power of sex to propel you is known as the Woman as Temptress. The idea here is that while the woman would provide short-term gratification, the powerful urges could easily distract you from your greater purpose and mission.

This is not to say that women or sex are bad. Both are great, but your journey is about a higher level of understanding of self and not giving in to carnal urges before you achieve complete control of the life you want. That's what self-mastery is about. You need to control the drive for sex and temper it with the drive for love, the drive for improvement, and the decision to act in certain ways to achieve a higher level of self-actualization, rather than to compete with others and win a masochistic pissing contest. And because the temptation and power of sex are quite possibly the most powerful in all of life, once you are able to demonstrate your ability to understand and master those drives, any hurdle in life can be overcome.

Still not convinced that sex is as important as we say it is? Here's a quick quiz.

On a scale of 1 to 10, how good do you think you are in bed?

Put another way, if your previous sexual partners had to rate you, where would they put you?

We've asked 300 men these same two questions, and not one of them responded with less than an 8 on either one.

Either every person we interviewed is a stud, or this quiz is giving us an important piece of info about men: they need to think of themselves as sexually competent in order to feel competent as men. It's just how you define yourself.

* Sorry, Robb Wolf. No offense, bro, but we love pizza.

This isn't something to be embarrassed about. Yes—there are other factors that define who you are. How you treat people matters, whether you're a good father or influence makes a difference, and doing your best to be a good human being will always be important. But on a primal level—your subconscious drivers of masculinity are strength and virility. These are a direct reflection of your ability not only to produce a family but also to protect it.

We were born to procreate and protect. No one can deny this sociological reality. And these priorities stem from sex and your sex drive. It doesn't matter if you believe in evolution or creationism—sex drive and the ability to reproduce and expand your legacy (through children) are an area of pride, joy, confidence, and motivation.

THE UNKNOWN POWER OF SEX

Accepting that sex is important is essential; it means you recognize that it's an important part of life, of relationships, and on the highest psychological level, it's directly tied to building a more confident and successful self. Here's why: University of Chicago researchers discovered that sexual frustration—a lack of interest in sex—is growing. If you feel this issue, don't worry, you're not alone. Some studies show that up to 20 percent of men have a declining interest in sex.

In non-survey studies, the reasons listed for a lower sex drive are a powerful warning shot to your masculinity, and one that deserves your attention. In a study conducted in Massachusetts, a little more than 10 percent of men mentioned having a lower sex drive compared to what they feel is normal. Of those with a drop in libido, nearly 30 percent had subpar testosterone levels. In the scientific world, that's what we call statistically significant. In your terms: that's no coincidence.

That dwindling sex drive opens Pandora's box on your sex life. We found more studies than we'd care to share (thirty-seven, to be exact) that showed a relationship between less sex and more stress. (On the flip side, the more sex you have, the less stress you experience.) Here's where performance anxiety takes a nasty turn.

As we've mentioned, stress increases your cortisol levels. Doctors have linked nearly every kind of stress to an increase in cortisol levels—and that includes illness, major life changes (such as losing a job or experiencing marital problems), and even nervousness and uncertainty. While we don't know the direct impact of how much those increases in cortisol affect your sex life, we do know that cortisol is kryptonite for your libido. So the more stress you have in your life, the more your sex life is suffering.

But new research from the University of Chicago is shedding light on just how significant cortisol can be in harming your sex life. In a study published in the *Journal of the American Medical Association,* men who slept fewer than five hours a night experienced a 15 percent drop in testosterone. And that drop was directly correlated to—and potentially caused by—an increase in cortisol. That might not seem like much, but these were twenty-four-year-old men who suddenly had the testosterone levels of someone fifteen years older.

The worst part? That's just *one week* of sleep deprivation. Imagine more. Or imagine that lack of sleep compounded with all the other stressors in your life.

Just in case you're not intimidated by that study, consider this fact: according to research published in the *Journal of Urology,* cortisol can literally kill the size of your erection. (Where were those studies when we were in college? Then again, we're sure we wouldn't really qualify.)

But that's only the beginning. And anytime a weak penis is the least of your problems, you've got some big fucking problems. When your stress becomes nonstop, it boosts cortisol levels to the point that you inhibit your body's main sex hormone: gonadotropin-releasing hormone (GnRH), say researchers at the University of California at Berkeley. That's a mouthful, but what you need to know is that lacking GnRH kills your drive for sexual activity and even weakens your sperm count, making it harder to reproduce. And while we're at it, it also increases your level of gonadotropin-inhibitory hormone (GnIH), which altogether kills your ability to reproduce.

And if that weren't enough, even if you were able to have get it up and have sex, the double dose of hormone shutdown could make it nearly impossible for you to have an orgasm.

Read that again: You. Can't. Orgasm.

How do you turn it all around? Like everything in this book, it starts with training. The right exercise prescription not only lowers your cortisol levels, but it also boosts your testosterone levels, giving you the sexual surge you need and want, say researchers from Turkey.

Remember, our goal is to provide quick fixes to the common problems that are unavoidable and ail all men. Our intent is twofold:

1. Make you aware of what's going on with your body so you give a shit.

2. Engineer your body so you can combat, defend, and overcome natural processes designed to make you less of a man. Most men fight blind. We want you to see clearly, be prepared, and defeat the enemy.

And that's why the training is about more than just stress. Or just muscle and fat loss. We're creating a body that, from the inside out, will make you the Alpha. Remember how we talked about how life doesn't work in a linear fashion? This is what we're talking about. Your stress might be *triggered* by life events, but it doesn't have to negatively affect your life. By following the steps to become an Alpha, you can prevent the problems that hold you back—whether they are related to stress, sleep, body fat, or anything else. Fix your hormones, improve your life.

Which brings us back to training. Researchers from Switzerland found that overweight men who exercised two and a half hours per week experienced a 46 percent decrease in hypogonadism. The name might sound cool, but it's actually a condition that is marked by low testosterone, low sex drive, and erectile dysfunction—also known as the holy trinity of the limp dick.

So we'll offer the type of exercise you need to set your body straight. Combine that with a diet that's high in fats, and you have a potent combination that will charge your sex hormones and counteract stress. The fat does the trick because testosterone is synthesized from cholesterol. Eat enough fat—but not too much (don't worry, we've taken care of the calculations for you in part 3)—and you'll increase your testosterone.

At the same time, you'll look more attractive, which will increases your self-perception of attractiveness, which will, in turn, make you more sexually confident, say University of Florida researchers. In fact, in the Florida study, participants who exercised felt just as confident about their appearance as those who had a fitter appearance. Meaning that the act of exercising itself improves self-perception and confidence. What's more, a University of Arkansas study found that 90 percent of men who rated their fitness level as above average found themselves more sexually desirable.

As you know, we're not about facades or smoke and mirrors. We will make you look better. But even if you want to deny the changes in the mirror (we're not sure why you would), this program will help you become more desirable. How? Because survey after survey, women say that the more sexual confidence you have, the more you are perceived as desirable.

Now, in case you have any question about it, we're about to prove that your sex drive really is the key to an unreal life.

MAKING THE LEAP: FROM SEX DRIVE TO SUCCESS

We've already established why improving your sex drive is important to your sex life. But the reason we care so much about your sex life is that it's integral to your ability to achieve success in other areas of your life. Freud was famous for theorizing about the psychological concept of sublimation. This theory stated that powerful impulses—such as sex—could be readily transformed into powerful socially accepted behaviors like becoming a better, more efficient worker. These hormonal drives were so powerful that they could be easily channeled into other areas, and they were a prominent driver of confidence and motivation.

Put another way, questions about your sex drive on an internal level cause fractures in self-confidence and negatively impact you in other areas of your life *without* your awareness.

This isn't what you'll list on a questionnaire or what you tell your boys at the bar. These are the questions that you only admit to yourself when you're alone. These are the thoughts that we know ruminate in your head.

We know you have them because we've had them too and so have all of our clients. You question if you're good enough. Are you attractive enough? Is there a reason you don't want sex more often? You might even question if your dick is big enough. You can't tell us that these questions—on issues that are so important to you—can't make you less confident in other areas of your life.

Or maybe more accurately worded—that being supremely confident on all of these issues can't increase your confidence in other aspects of your life. According to researchers at the University of Chicago, only 23 percent of men who have a loss of libido still feel content with their lives. The study examined how often men think about sex. While survey data was collected, the researchers made some very interesting conclusions. They felt that the stats would have been even more staggering but that, for many men, the thought of not being sexually active was *normal*.

We're not sure which is more troubling—the drop in libido or the idea that men aren't bothered by this decrease.

Although women with lower libido tend to experience higher levels of happiness, men aren't wired that way. For men, sex drive is more closely linked to self-concept, and thus it has a greater impact on confidence and enjoyment of *all* activities, say the study authors.

At this point, it really shouldn't be a surprise. Remember, confidence breeds confidence. Success breeds success. It's why we know that changing your body will start this transformation. But in order to create an unreal life, your physical transformation must lead to a sexual metamorphosis.

In the end, when everything is equal, your success and your happiness are directly linked to your confidence. And the strongest psychological determinant of confidence is—you guessed it—your physical and sexual presence.

ELEVEN WAYS TO BOOST YOUR SEX DRIVE

This book is not about showing you the techniques to be a better lover. We leave that for other people and more hands-on experience. But we do want to help you fight off all the elements that are killing your sex drive and making it harder to establish your confidence. So we identified the problems that are killing your hormones and your ability to have the type of sex life you want. And the type of sex life that doesn't have to dwindle.

Lose Your Gut

Listen, we have nothing against fat people. But it's a proven fact that people who don't like the way they look have less sex. It's tied to psychological and cognitive deficiencies on many levels. To start, you don't feel attractive, which creates stress and lowers sex drive. This lowered sex drive causes you to have sex less frequently, which forces a sense of learned helplessness. That is, you don't think you'll have sex again, so there's no reason to try. Or if you're married, it means that you stop instigating sex the way you did earlier in the relationship. It's a vicious and dangerous cycle for your body and your relationship.

All the while, your excess fat is brewing up a physiological storm that is waging war on your sex drive. According to a study published in the journal *Endocrinology*, the more fat you carry, the lower the testosterone production. After all, the genes that control your testosterone levels also control your body fat. They are directly linked, and therefore more body fat means less testosterone. And the less testosterone you have, the lower your libido. If that wasn't bad enough, as your fat levels increase, so do your estrogen levels. And according to Spanish researchers, once your estrogen levels get too high, you can kiss your sex life good-bye.

Lift Heavy Weights

As you know, we're fitness professionals. So now might be a good time to remind you that our professional status doesn't mean we only know how to build muscle and burn fat. We also understand how lifting weights can completely change your physiology so you function like a different human being.

So please trust us when we tell you this: lifting weights *will* improve your sex life. Not *might* or *maybe*. It will happen.

Lifting weights increases GH and testosterone—in a big way. Finnish researchers found that guys who regularly lift free weights (like dumbbells and barbells) boost their testosterone levels by up to 49 percent. And that testosterone increase is directly linked to more sexual virility.

So pumping iron boosts your libido. But that's no reason to think it can save your sex life, right?

Wrong.

Most men (and doctors) had assumed for decades that your sex life naturally declines as you age. After all, you already know that GH and testosterone start to drop after the age of thirty. And that's why everything becomes a little softer. But when it comes to your sex life, new research has found that it's not aging that reduces your testosterone and subsequently your sex drive. It's inactivity. Australian researchers recently discovered that the drop in testosterone wasn't correlated with age but rather with behaviors such as obesity, low activity levels, and smoking.

That means lifestyle decisions that cause poor health are killing your sex life. The insulin resistance. The extra fat. The cortisol building. Since most people become less active as they grow older, their testosterone levels drop—and with it so does their sexual mojo. But if you stay active, the decrease of testosterone between the ages of forty and eighty can be almost completely blunted. Add it to the list of ways the iron game keeps you strong.

Eat More Fat

By now you know that eating more fat is not the demonized cause of obesity that many people think it is. You need fat to lose fat. You need fat to build muscle. And guess what? You also need fat to have awesome sex. Fat plays an important role in regulating all your sex hormones. And fats are integral to your sexual functioning. British scientists discovered that having productive, fertile sperm depends on polyunsaturated fats, which you can receive from fatty fish (like salmon or trout) or fish oil supplements. Those same fats also promote good circulation and blood flow. If you weren't aware, your erection depends on healthy blood flow, meaning that without those healthy fats, buildup can occur in your arteries that will hurt your sexual health.

Want more proof? Vegetarians—whose diets are typically lower in fat—were found to have lower levels of testosterone compared to those who had higher fat intake in their diet, according to the *Journal of Endocrinology* and the *American Journal of Clinical Nutrition*. Is that a definitive cause-and-effect relationship? Of course not. But it is a powerful correlation that shouldn't be overlooked when you consider the hormonal benefits of fat and the links between fat intake and improved sexual functioning.

A quick warning: do all you can to avoid trans fats. They can potentially hurt the quality of your sperm. Trans fats are the reason fat has such a bad rap. They are artificially produced fats that are linked to every possible disease, and they will make your gut expand faster than you can say, "Doughnuts." Trans fats exist in many processed foods like cookies, fries, chips, and muffins.

The bottom line: Fat doesn't make you fat. But the wrong *type* of fat can do damage.

Eat Less Soy

When we say to eat less soy, what we really mean is that you should stop eating all soy. We don't care if you're vegetarian or vegan or you run a soy farm. Soy is not good for men. And that's not only our opinion. The brilliant minds at Harvard found a strong relationship between poor sperm quality and erectile dysfunction and the amount of soy in a man's diet.

Soy is great for women (in moderation) because it has estrogenic effects. But as we mentioned before, as you build estrogen, you simultaneously kill your sex dive.

The hard part about cutting soy is that it's hiding in lots of products that you probably think are harmless, including protein powders and bars, and many cereal products. Vegetarians typically have diets that are higher in soy, which might be another reason (in addition to fat intake) why vegetarians have been found to have lower levels of testosterone.

In order to avoid the dangerous bean, it might suit you best to check the food label twice before you inadvertently fill your body with a substance that will slowly but surely turn you into more of a woman. No joke.

Be a Strategic Drinker (Translation: Drink Less Beer)

Cheat days are an important part of our fitness plan, and one of our favorite ways to cheat (especially during the fall) is to go crazy on Sunday. What better way to enjoy the NFL than with pizza, beer, and wings? We can't think of a better way to be gluttonous without getting fat.

But if there's one element we want you to be wary of, it's the beer. That's right, not the pizza or the wings. For that matter, we're not too worried about cheesecake, pie, or even doughnut ice cream sandwiches.* That's because alcohol has a negative impact on your testosterone levels. More specifically, Dutch researchers found that any regular alcoholic consumption can drop your testosterone levels nearly 10 percent and that the associated drop is linked to a decrease in sex drive.

What's worse, we're not talking about the impact of drinking over an extended period of time. The scientists found the drop to occur in just three weeks' time, meaning prolonged drinking could have an even more dramatic impact. And then there's the impact you can't even see. Alcohol is very easily oxidized in your body. Without getting too technical, oxidized stress is not good for your sex life. It can damage the DNA of your sperm and decrease your sperm count, making it harder for you to procreate.

Not to mention, while having whiskey dick might help you last longer, inevitably it decreases sensitivity and sexual enjoyment. And if sex isn't enjoyable, well then you're kind of missing the point.

Again, the goal is not to avoid drinking; it's just to drink less overall. And when you do drink, the goal should be less beer—except for on a football Sunday. Instead, go for a glass or two of wine if you want to take the edge off after a long workday.

Set Your Alarm an Hour Earlier

Raise your hand if you've ever started your morning with an erection.

---

* A *doughnut ice cream sandwich* is a real thing; essentially, a doughnut is sliced in half lengthwise and two to three scoops of ice cream and a few toppings are placed on the bottom half. The top half is covered with traditional donut frosting and more toppings, then placed on the ice cream. Bam—ice cream all up in your doughnut. They probably serve them at a lot of places across the country, but the one we're familiar with is the cleverly named Holey Cream, located in Hell's Kitchen. If you're ever in NYC on your cheat day, stop in and tell 'em we sent you.

Okay, know that we're all in this together, here's what you need to know: you need to start loving morning sex. We don't care if you're tired or your wife / partner / one-night stand doesn't feel sexy in the morning. Your testosterone levels peak in the morning. It's why your dick wakes up packing more power than a box of Viagra. And what happens when you have sex? You experience a beneficial surge of testosterone.

Listen, you need to view yourself like a coach of your body. And a good coach puts his team in the right situations for success. Just as you need to find the ideal times and frequency to eat, you should also be having sex when your body is primed to do so.

If you're noticing that you're having less sex, the easiest solution is simply to set your alarm an hour earlier. (But don't get less sleep; adjust when you go to bed.) Most people don't have morning sex because they don't feel they have time. And most people don't have night sex because they're ready to sleep. By setting the alarm an hour earlier, you remove both of these problems, and you take advantage of the most enjoyable way to improve your hormones.

Eat Less Sugar (Or Eat More Sugar at the Right Times)

When it comes to sugar, there are two adages that will help you determine how to navigate your consumption: When you want to eat it, remember that a little can go a long way. When you're wondering if you've had too much, remember: everything in moderation.

For us, *moderation* tends to mean one day a week when you binge on the stereotypical "bad" sugars. Otherwise, it's best to limit sugars for the very reasons you expect—they're not good for your health, and they make you fat. But too much sugar can also punish your sex life. A study in the *Journal of Sexual Medicine* discovered that healthier blood sugar levels improve your sexual health. And by sexual health, we mean more desire to fuck and less erectile dysfunction.

Sugar plays a dangerous role with insulin. Specifically, taking in too much sugar on a consistent basis increases insulin resistance. As you know, you *don't* want to be insulin resistant; in addition to all the negative attributes we've already described, insulin resistance impairs vasodilation—otherwise known as blood flow—by clogging your artery walls. That decrease in blood flow is all it takes to weaken your erections as well as to potentially cause health problems in your nether regions. And no one wants problems down there.

In terms of sugars that are okay, you don't need to spend much time stressing about fruits. Instead, watch out for all the hidden sugars in packaged foods, and be wary of taking in too much dried fruit or juice. We wouldn't recommend having either more than once or twice a week, and just a serving at that. You'd be surprised what one glass of juice per day could do to your blood sugar levels.

Watch Less Porn

For every guy who ever claimed that watching porn was merely for research, you've officially been liberated. There's some serious science behind watching porn, but that's not a good thing if you've made erotica a frequent hobby. According to research published in *Psychology Today*, watching porn can cause neurochemical changes that kill your ability to become aroused.

The power player behind this phenomenon is dopamine. You might know dopamine as the neurotransmitter in your brain that influences your ability to feel and experience pleasure. Not surprisingly, when you watch porn, it triggers a strong dopamine reaction. This is a good thing. But it becomes bad when you constantly or repeatedly create a dopamine surge from watching porn. Like any drug, you become resistant. In this case, that means you desensitize your ability to become aroused by sex and other pleasurable experiences.

This is a very dangerous situation. Too much porn can literally decrease your ability to form intimate relationships, and regular sex will no longer be enjoyable. This has been shown to make people withdraw entirely from actual sex and instead search for more outlandish forms of pornography that might trigger dopamine and cause them to experience arousal.

What this means is your boundaries will be pushed so far that it'll be difficult to be aroused by anything basic. Over a long enough period of time, the extended exposure will make it harder for the act of sex to get you aroused.

While we're not saying you shouldn't watch porn, we are saying that you want to be mindful that it can have a detrimental effect on your intimacy and arousal. As they always said at the end of *GI Joe*, "Knowing is half the battle."

Check Your Prescription Meds

There's a reason why depression is one of the biggest hurdles to sexual satisfaction. Once you become depressed, there's a dangerous catch-22 associated with finding your way out of the dark and into happiness. If you're depressed, some of the most effective drugs you can take are selective serotonin reuptake inhibitors (SSRIs). These drugs increase the amount of serotonin, another feel-good neurotransmitter. From a chemical standpoint, you almost have no choice but to feel better. There's just one catch—SSRIs also interfere with sexual pleasure. Some situations are so bad that SSRIs have been shown to inhibit your ability to orgasm. This, in turn, makes you feel bad and can increase symptoms of depression even when physiologically you have medicine that is supposed to make you happier.

Unfortunately, there's no simple fix for this situation. You have to experiment on a personal level. Researchers suggest starting with a low dosage to assess if your depression symptoms improve without any negative sexual consequences. But if your sex drive and pleasure disappear, it might be time for a different medical solution.

Get More Sleep

Are you starting to sense a theme in this book? Sleeping is incredibly important to many of the fundamental attributes of being a man—and that includes your sex life. The sweet spot appears to be five hours, say researchers at University of Chicago. (Remember, your *goal* is still six hours. But when you get less than five hours, that's when the worst consequences appear to take over.) That's the breaking point where your testosterone levels drop. And like booze, it doesn't take long to have a significant impact. Just one week of sleeping less than five hours a night can drop your levels to those of someone fifteen years older. That's significant when you consider that testosterone has been shown to drop up to 1 percent every year after you hit thirty. The men in the study reported that the drop in sleep quality resulted in less happiness, satisfaction, and sex drive.

A requirement should then be to get *at least* six hours of sleep per night, and when you think about it, that's not a big request. If you struggle sleeping, here are a few tricks that might help:

1. **Make your room colder.** This improves your ability to fall asleep.

2. **Eat more carbs late at night.** We already told you that you should be having carbs at night because it's good for your body and your workouts, but the carbs will also help you pass out. Need proof? Think about every Thanksgiving after you eat approximately two pounds of stuffing and sweet potatoes. We'll show you how many carbs to eat at night, but in general, you'll be splitting all your carbs between two meals: after your workout and before bed. If you work out late at night, then prepare yourself for an evening carb party!

3. **Eat protein before bed.** When you're throwing down your carbs, make sure you're combining them with some protein. It can be a chicken breast or just a scoop of protein powder. Protein contains amino acids, one of which is L-tryptophan. If you love *Seinfeld*, you already know this as the secret sauce in turkey that makes people tired. Your brain uses tryptophan to produce melatonin and serotonin, both of which improve your sleep.

4. **Have a cheat day.** That's right. Here's another reason why cheat days are so great—low leptin levels can hurt your sleep. So by going higher carb, you'll bump up your leptin and improve your quality of sleep.

5. **Sleep in a dark room.** This might seem obvious, but your sleep cycle is dependent on circadian rhythms. In other words, when it's light your body "knows" to be awake, and when it's dark it makes you want to sleep. The light decreases melatonin production, which makes it harder for you to go to sleep.

6. **Avoid caffeine before you sleep.** Another no-brainer, but even if you don't feel that caffeine has an impact on you, it's still a stimulant. Since the half-life of caffeine can be a while, depending on the individual, we recommend that you avoid caffeine after four P.M. if possible.*

* We admit that while writing this book, we violated this rule. A lot. And it kept us up, which was a good thing for finishing the book but a bad thing for our sleep and our sex lives.

Take More Vacations

We've already made it perfectly clear that stress harms your hormones in a way that is frighteningly dangerous for your sex drive. And while it'd be great to live a life that's free of stress (in fact, it's one of our primary goals for this book), we know it might take some time to progress to that level. So as you learn the ropes, your easiest solution is to take a vacation.

A nine-year study found that vacations are one of the best stress relievers. They're so powerful that men who take vacations have lower levels of cortisol and are 30 percent less likely to die from heart disease. The key wasn't the length of the vacation, but rather the frequency. It's a good reminder that if you play and work hard, you need consistent tune-ups to keep you performing at a high level. In that way, your body is like a car. If you drive it all the time and only bring it in once per year, your car will die on you sooner than you want.

We know that vacations are a luxury, but a getaway can occur in many forms. And because price shouldn't be a limiting factor that prevents you from getting away, we recommend the Alpha vacation. Go camping, hiking, or kayaking or spend a night sleeping in a tent somewhere. The idea is that you unplug, get away, and include some sort of exercise. (Bonus points if you do pull-ups in the trees.) Bring your guy friends and enjoy a weekend. The stress that will be removed by this type of approach will shock you. A few days every few months can literally make a difference that could help you live longer.

CONFIDENCE

We don't need to tell you that sex feels good. But there's another psychological benefit of sex that plays an important role in your development as a man. Sex allows you to feel that you have fulfilled a biological imperative in that you've taken steps toward procreation; this satisfies the ego on a deeply subconscious level.

When you fulfill your ego on a subconscious level, it bubbles up to the conscious level. We probably don't have to explain this to you. Any time you start having more sex—especially with someone new—you walk with a little more spring in your step. Of course this is partially due to the fact that sex is fucking awesome. But, more than anything else, sex has reaffirmed—or created—an unwavering belief that you can accomplish anything. It is acceptance and approval at the highest level; it's the most visceral form of approval. Someone is literally letting you *in* to their body.

Acknowledging that your confidence is tied in part to your sex life, and in particular how active and successful it is, does not mean you are drawing all your self-worth from your sexual accomplishments. It just means that you acknowledge that you're human, and more importantly, a man.

A true Alpha accepts these things and makes them part of who he is. He realizes that understanding the relationship between sex and confidence gives him power over himself. It allows him to objectively look at his self-esteem in times when his sex life is not active; this knowledge allows him to understand that the reason he's feeling down may be due in part to the lack of sex.

All of that creates a greater control over your sense of self. You'll be able to objectively monitor how you're feeling.

On the other hand, in times of your life when you're having sexual success—with one or many partners—the Alpha awareness of the relationship between sex and confidence will ensure that you don't turn into a cocky asshole who thinks he can bang the entire world just because he's having a lot of sex.

But remember, sex is just a catalyst. The bigger picture is how you build confidence, in general. The easiest and most *powerful* ways to do that are by improving your physical attributes through exercise and diet, and by boosting your sex drive.

Once you experience that success, you'll learn to link your confidence to other things. After all, in order to hit your target, you must first learn how to pull the trigger—by optimizing your hormones and experiencing those benefits—and then you can look for more bullets. As you build confidence, this more readily allows you to take a more honest appraisal of your self-worth so you can look at all the things you have to offer and how they can drive or further boost your confidence.

As we stated in the Alpha Traits, a true Alpha is confident but not cocky. He has a very real understanding of what he can and can't do. However, the Alpha's confidence is high because of his assessment of his abilities, and thus he realizes there isn't much he can't do.

HAPPINESS

Take a moment to think about the last time you were happy. We're not talking about the fleeting moments when you smile and laugh. We mean *real* happiness. A permanent state of being when you were content with yourself and the world you live in and you didn't experience any stress or desire for anything more.

For some people, this type of fantasy is reserved for sleep. Stress is a part of life. Frustration is inevitable. And in a world where what you can achieve appears limited by what you directly control, it's inevitable that you're always going to want more.

Or is it?

As sex is a catalyst for confidence, happiness is a by-product of creating more control in your life. This doesn't mean building a world where you are insulated and every person and decision is a puppet that creates a safe environment. This is about using your newfound confidence to establish more comfort in your universe, which allows you to stress less and stop worrying about everything that corrupts your happiness.

ENGINEERING THE ALPHA

SUBJECT: *Josh Hamilton*

THE ORDINARY WORLD

I'm the guy who loves the fitness industry. I read articles. Have always been considered "fit" and would love to make this my career. But the fitness industry was frustrating. On one hand, quality information is available at the flick of a finger and has brought joy, strength, and muscle to many individuals, changing their lives for the better. At the same time, the plethora of information can oftentimes be so confusing and frustrating that it pushes you away from fitness and makes you see no hope for improvement. That was my experience. I had a strong desire to better myself, and the quest for physique enhancement became my obsession, but one that ended up tearing at the integrity of my social and family life.

ACCEPTING THE CALL

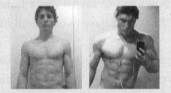 *Purging through misinformation was an arduous battle, but the need to educate myself properly and surround myself with incredible people prevailed when I found Roman. He played an integral role in my physical, social, and intellectual transformation. He helped me improve and sharpen my mind-set, values, goals, outlook, and physique. This transformation marked much more than simply adding pounds of muscle to my frame; it signified a new chapter of my life.*

ALPHA STATUS

Radically changing my physique has solidified my shift as a man. My body now represents what I am capable of achieving and is my foundation for success and growth. After the program, I gained the courage to move across the country alone to further my education and improve my environment, started my own business, radically increased my level of confidence, and started going after my lifelong dreams. The looks, smiles, and groping from women are all positives, even for a guy that didn't have much trouble with the vixens. The skill of critical thinking and trying to improve myself to better the world is one of the most valuable and life-changing lessons I'll ever receive.

HOW TO TAKE CONTROL OF YOUR LIFE

Once you start to execute control with any level of regularity, you no longer have time to focus on the things you can't control. Once you get into the habit of making sure you have your umbrella, you stop worrying if it's going to rain. This clears your mind. This allows you to make decisions more clearly, which helps you make better decisions. Your field of vision narrows, your focus improves, and your mind will be *like water.**

Remember, success is a learned habit. So once you get in the habit of trusting your decisions, it becomes easier to make decisions more clearly. So how do you start the process?

It starts with the gym. It might sound ridiculous, shallow, and superficial. And on some level, it is. But there are few things in life that you can *directly* influence as much as your performance in the gym. It's superficial to think that squats, deadlifts, and pull-ups can bring you to a place where you feel happy; but it's not that far out of reach. Cornell University researchers established that the more control you feel in your life, the more likely you are to be happy. And in the gym, you are in control. It doesn't matter where you start, what you look like, or your ultimate goal. You control whether you do the work or not and whether you eat the right foods at the right times—you possess the power to turn your body into an object of desire and a beacon of confidence.

And while we are the ones guiding you, you're still the one making the decision to act. You're the one visiting the gym. You're the one following the diet. You're the one making the decision to be productive. And ultimately, you'll become the hero and be able to walk on your own with success in your back pocket.

As Henry Rollins said, "There is no better way to fight weakness than with strength."

So start with that decision: to learn control over your body and your mind. Then you'll experience the control and the resulting happiness that inevitably comes when you make the right choice *consistently.* That's the key. Success isn't meant to be an aberration. Anyone can have success once—and rarely are those people happy. Happiness is a state of being, not a temporary goal or a fleeting desire.

So you must practice the habits we share in this book as a routine. All of this will become much clearer once you start the actual routine. We feel that understanding the *why* of engineering the Alpha is the most important element that will allow you to see the program to the end and experience all the benefits of becoming the Alpha. And don't worry, there's much more flexibility than you might think in this program. But your decisions—specifically the choice to commit—are what will allow you to feel better about yourself.

Your hormones will be optimized, and your brain will function better. Your body will function at a higher level than you thought possible. And suddenly you'll be more confident in your ability to create change.

* We stole this from Bruce Lee. Simple and brilliant.

That's when you can start translating your control to other areas of life. The workplace is a great example. Optimizing your hormones will make you smarter and more competent. You'll think clearer and become more efficient. But the biggest difference will be the confidence in yourself and the decisions you make. Scaling the corporate ladder is not about being the smartest guy in the room; it's about making the best decisions. And those better decisions will occur with better confidence, more focus and clarity, and less self-doubt—all of which derives from *other* areas of your life.

THE MAN'S GUIDE TO NUTRITION

WARNING: *Read this* carefully. *We have crammed in a lot of information about the types of foods you'll be eating. In many ways, this might be one of the most important chapters because guys are notoriously bad at following diets. We hate the d-word because a diet is really just how you eat. And since everyone has a way of eating,* dieting *is usually an unfairly negative term.*

That said, food is a foundational component of hormone optimization, and therefore what you eat is an essential part of engineering the Alpha. We're going to talk about nutrition here, but this is not *the exact program. So put away your pen and paper, shut down your note-taking app, and continue reading leisurely. Every single detail will be found in part 3, including a customized formula that you'll use for every phase in the program.*

That said, if you want to get started immediately and can't wait to see what's in the plan, flip ahead to that part and enjoy.

At the same time, know that we created this section for a reason: we want you to understand why *you're eating what you are so that you can make your own good decisions. That's part of how you'll be able to gain control and be an Alpha. The more educated you are, the less frustration you'll experience, the more control you'll have, and the better you'll look and feel.*

Now that we're on the same page, we've provided a primer on what you need to know about macronutrients—or more specifically carbohydrates, proteins, and fats. Arm yourself with this information and no food marketer will ever fool you again. Even better? You'll know how to take advantage of food so you can strategically eat all the stuff you love and still look fucking amazing.

■ CARBOHYDRATES

Carbohydrates seem to be the focus of most diets you read about (especially fat-loss diets), so it makes sense to start here. Carbs have taken a real beating in the media ever since some guy named Atkins (you may have heard of him) decided we weren't allowed to eat doughnuts anymore. (Prior to this we were allowed to eat doughnuts, but they had to be reduced fat; this made us feel better about ourselves.)

All joking aside, carbs do get kind of a bad rap, or at least a worse one than they deserve. Carbs come in a variety of forms. Some are good for you, and some are bad. The bad ones are usually highly processed and could barely be considered food other than the fact that they're edible. They may be delicious, but they're also the result of some crazy scientific processes.

Of course, if you process the crap out of anything, it reaches a point where it just isn't healthy anymore. This doesn't mean carbs are evil and to blame for all the ills of the world from the Nazis to the obesity epidemic—it just means processed foods are great at making people fat.

Anyway, carbohydrates are made up of sugar molecules, which your body breaks down into fuel, especially when you're working hard. Sugars, starches, and fiber are all basic forms of the carbohydrate.

There are two main types of carbohydrates: simple and complex.*

Simple Carbohydrates

In the most basic sense, simple carbohydrates include table sugar, syrup, and soda. Most of the time, these carbs should be avoided (exceptions include cheat days) and are usually the "bad carbs" that fitness pros talk about. Also included on this list are things like candy, snuggles, cake, beer, puppies, cookies, fun, and unicorn magic. In other words, the best ones.**

Complex Carbohydrates

Complex carbohydrates include oatmeal, apples, cardboard, and peas.

For a long time, people believed that complex carbohydrates were universally better for you than simple carbohydrates, but that isn't always the case.

You see, your body takes both complex and simple carbohydrates and tries to break them down into useable sugar energy to fuel your muscles and organs. It's not the type of carbohydrate that really matters, but how quickly your body can break it down and how much it will spike your blood glucose levels.

It's not as simple as dividing complex carbs from simple ones, though. A slightly more sophisticated way to rate carbohydrate quality is something called the glycemic index (GI). The GI attempts to classify foods by how quickly they break down and how high they boost blood sugar levels.

---

* We could also mention fibrous carbs that you can find in foods like green veggies, lettuce, cabbage, broccoli, sprouts, spinach, cauliflower, peppers, cucumbers, zucchini . . . buuuut we won't. For the purposes of this discussion of carbs, we only want to touch on stuff that counts. We usually don't recommend counting calories (or carbs for that matter) coming from fibrous carbs. This doesn't mean that these foods don't count. They do. But we've never met anyone who got fat eating too many vegetables. And after coaching literally thousands of people, we've determined that eating more veggies has always been a good thing.

** Minor homage to Superbad.

WHAT IS LEAN BODY MASS?

LBM is the amount of muscle you have on your body. To figure out your LBM, just use this three-step process:

1. Figure out your body fat percentage.

2. Subtract your body fat percentage from 100. This is your fat-free mass.

3. Multiply your fat-free mass (as a percentage) by your body weight. This result is your LBM.

So let's say you're a 200-pound man with 20 percent body fat.

1. You're 20% body fat.

2. 100 − 20 = 80% fat-free mass.

3. 200 pounds x 0.8 = 160 pounds.

Your LBM is 160. As your percentage of body fat changes, so will your LBM.

We will refer to LBM in several places throughout the book, so keep this formula in mind. Or write it down. Or tear out this page. It's your book, so the choice is yours.

For a while, the GI was all the rage, and people argued that by following a low-GI diet, you'd keep insulin levels in check even while eating more carbs overall. This has turned out to be only partially true. Which is to say that while it's probably better to eat low-GI foods than high ones, there probably won't be a tremendous difference in your waistline if you're still eating your weight in sweet potatoes instead of Cheerios.

Neither low-carb diets nor low-GI diets are a magic pill for fat loss; the main thing is to eat the right amount of healthy foods that fuel metabolism, which in turn will help you burn fat.

The important thing to remember is that your body needs carbs, even if some of the fad diets tell you otherwise. Without carbohydrates, your body will begin to break down your muscle tissue to fuel your body, which will sabotage your efforts.

Carb lovers lament low-carb diets, and anti-carb crusaders posit that you can avoid carbs for the most part and still do well. The truth is a bit of middle ground. So yes, speaking generally you should avoid simple carbs and high-GI foods, but that doesn't mean you can eat complex carbs or low-GI foods all day either.

We do not think that carbs are the devil; however, we find that our clients do better in terms of fat loss on low(er) carbs. But low carbs does not mean no carbs. As a general rule, we like to set daily carbohydrate intake at around 0.5 to 0.75 grams per pound of lean body mass (LBM).

Most importantly, the problem with carbs is eating them alone. Instead, you should try to have carbs with protein. Eating carbs and protein together slows the rate of digestion of the carbs, lowers the glycemic/insulin response, and can generally offset some of the negatives that come with carbohydrate consumption.

■ FATS

For a long time, fats were like carbs—blamed for every damn health problem possible. It's the reason that for nearly twenty years, low fat *was synonymous with* healthy. *And for many people—maybe even several of you reading this—that's still how you determine whether something is safe to eat. If it's low fat, it has to be good. Or if it doesn't have saturated fat, then it's okay.*

Lies piled on top of more lies. As our nation's fat consumption decreased, its obesity increased, according to CDC data. This was due to a variety of factors—the frequency of meals and snacks, the size of meals, and the consumption of sugar.

So what is the bottom line on fat? For starters, it's a necessary component of your diet and something you're probably not consuming enough of. Fat is good. It's good for testosterone. It's good for your heart (yes, you read that correctly). And it's good for your muscles.

Fat plays an important role in helping the general functioning of your body. Fat is a critical coating for nerves. This coating serves to speed up conduction down the nerve so that every time a neurochemical signal is sent through your body (any time your brain wants to tell your body to do something), it happens efficiently.

Fat also serves as a substrate for a whole set of hormones known as eicosanoids. While we're bordering on becoming too geeky, eicosanoids are essential for numerous functions that regulate things like blood pressure, inflammation, and even blood clotting. This kind of fat is needed for basic human physiology, which is reason enough to include it in your diet.

Now that you know why fats are needed in your diet, here's what you should know about the different types of fats—and why each needs to be included in your diet, with the exception of trans fats.

Monounsaturated Fats

Monounsaturated fats are found mostly in high-fat fruits such as avocados as well as nuts like pistachios, almonds, walnuts, and cashews. This type of fat can also be found in olive oil.

Monounsaturated fats help lower bad cholesterol and raise good cholesterol. They've also been proven to help fight weight gain and may even help reduce body fat levels.

Polyunsaturated Fats

Like monounsaturated fats, these good fats help fight bad cholesterol. Polyunsaturated fats stay liquid even in the cold because their melting point is lower than that of monounsaturated fats.

You can find polyunsaturated fats in foods like salmon, fish oil, sunflower oil, seeds, and soy. Polyunsaturated fats contain omega-3 and omega-6 fatty acids, which have largely been processed out of our food.

Omega-3s and 6s are very important and are oftentimes referred to as essential fatty acids, or EFAs. These cannot be manufactured by our bodies, and so it becomes essential to ingest them. And because your body needs these sources to function optimally and remain healthy, it's your job to make sure your diet has enough of these fats to avoid problems and breakdown.

Saturated Fats

Saturated fats might be the most misunderstood substance you can eat. And for good reason: there have been studies linking high intake of saturated fats to heart disease.

The idea that saturated fats have been proven to be anything other than delicious goes back to a pretty flawed research study from the 1950s in which a scientist named Ancel Keys published a paper that laid the blame for the worldwide heart disease increase on dietary fat intake.

However, there were major flaws to his study. For one, in his conclusions he only used data from a small portion of the countries where data was available on fat consumption versus heart disease death rate. When researches have gone back in and looked at the data from all the countries where data was available, there actually was no link between fat consumption and heart disease deaths. In retrospect, it seems that Keys jumped the gun here and landed on conclusions that didn't really have a basis in fact.

In a more modern-day context, books like The China Study and movies like Forks Over Knives have pointed the finger at saturated fats—and all animal fats—as the reason for all health problems. And yet, these studies all took a very slanted bias toward the saturated fat hypothesis and completely ignored populations that were incredibly healthy despite diets based on saturated fats. In fact, people who live in Tokelau (a territory off of New Zealand) eat a diet that is 50 percent saturated fats, and they have cardiovascular health superior to any other group of people, and yet this data and information is ignored.

Now, this book is not about debunking The China Study, *but it is important that that information be thoroughly criticized and debunked. If it were accurate, we would support it. We don't have a horse in the diet race other than to help people live and eat in the best way possible and live longer, more fulfilled lives.*

Listen, we don't mind admitting when we are wrong. Ten years ago we were both wrong about saturated fats, just as we were wrong about how many meals you should eat per day. That's why we spent so much time going through all the research, testing out thousands of clients, and then coming to you with information that we knew would benefit you. And in part 3, we're going to provide meal plans, preferred food options, and even personalized calculations that will allow you to know exactly what you need to be eating to become the Alpha.

And our conclusions—supported by science—are that your diet should include saturated fats and you shouldn't stress about the quantity. There are several studies of hunter-gatherer tribes that consumed 50 to 70 percent of all their calories from saturated fats without any health problems. When you receive the specific calculations for your fat intake, up to half of the fat can derive from saturated fats.

Even Walter Willett, chairman of the Department of Nutrition at Harvard, has publicly stated (after a twenty-year review of research) that fats—and more specifically saturated fats—are not the cause of the obesity crisis and are not the cause of heart disease.

Saturated fats also get a bit of a bad rap because they have been shown to elicit and increase cholesterol in the bloodstream. Again, we have to say that this is not as scary as the media makes it seem—cholesterol concerns are highly overblown. The truth is, cholesterol actually acts as an antioxidant against dangerous free radicals within the blood.

When there are high levels of undesirable substances in the blood (caused by the dietary intake of damaged fats, highly processed foods, and large quantities of sugars), cholesterol levels rise in order to combat these substances.

Further to that, cholesterol is also necessary for the production of a number of hormones, some of which help fight against heart disease. Somewhat more cogent to our purposes in this book is the fact that cholesterol is the direct precursor to all sex hormones—including testosterone. In other words, the higher your cholesterol is, the higher your testosterone is likely to be.

Listen, saturated fat is one of the best sources of energy for your body. It's why your body naturally stores carbohydrates as saturated fat. Are you going to argue with one of the most basic structures of how your body was intended to work? Not to mention, saturated fats are some of the most satiating foods, meaning they keep you fuller longer. And research shows diets that are higher in saturated fats are oftentimes lower in total calories consumed. And, as we alluded to already, saturated fats boost testosterone, which as we've already mentioned about a hundred times, is what makes you a man.

That leaves you with one option: assuming you're not a vegetarian, you should be eating red meat, dairy, and eggs to consume your share of saturated fats.

Trans Fats

Trans fats are the black sheep of the fat family. Trans fats are the worst fats, and in truth, one of the worst forms of food that you could possibly consume. They're found in foods such as French fries, potato chips, and most fried foods.

While some trace amounts of trans fats are naturally occurring in meats and other foods, by and large, most are not naturally occurring. Instead, they are generally manmade.

Trans fats are made by a chemical process called partial hydrogenation. Manufacturers take liquid vegetable oil (an otherwise decent monounsaturated fat) and pack it with hydrogen atoms, which convert it into a solid fat. This makes what seems to be an ideal fat for the food industry because it has a high melting point and a smooth texture, and it can be reused in deep-fat frying.

Essentially, trans fats come about as a result of overprocessing our foods in order to offer consumers a longer shelf life. If your food is pre-packaged, it's a pretty safe bet that it has its fair share of trans fats. If you are serious about your goals, you should try to avoid trans fats at all costs. Or if you just don't want to be eating plastic garbage.

Of course, we take a moderate approach. If you're limiting your intake of junk foods, exercising regularly, and getting good nutrition otherwise—including a variety of healthy fats—then chances are, you can have the occasional Twinkie once every few months and be okay.

■ PROTEIN

While both carbs and fats have spent their time as public enemy #1, being demonized or lauded by turns, no macronutrient has enjoyed the rise to prominence and popularity as much as our friend, protein.

A favorite among bodybuilders, athletes, and just about any fitness enthusiast, protein is used by your body to repair damaged muscle, bone, skin, teeth, and hair, among other things. Think of it as the mortar between the bricks; without it, the entire structure of your body begins to break down.

Protein helps to create an anabolic hormonal environment (good for muscle building and fat loss), and along the lines of the brick metaphor, it provides a lot of the materials used to build your muscles.

There are two categories of protein: complete and incomplete. Protein is comprised of smaller molecules called amino acids. There are twenty-two amino acids that warrant attention, of which nine belong to a subcategory that can only be obtained through your food. Your body can manufacture the remainder of the amino acids.

The nine amino acids that can only be obtained from the food you eat are called essential amino acids. For those interested in such things, the essential amino acids are:

Tryptophan	**Phenylalanine**	**Leucine**
Lysine	**Threonine**	**Histidine**
Methionine	**Valine**	**Isoleucine**

A complete protein (also known as a whole protein) is one that contains adequate portions of those nine amino acids. By contrast, an incomplete protein is one that is lacking in one or more of those amino acids.

These amino acids also help your body create hormones that help regulate things like blood pressure and blood sugar levels, which are directly responsible for your metabolic rate and muscular growth. In short, protein is extremely important, especially the complete proteins that are found in foods such as fish, poultry, eggs, red meat, and cheese.

VEGAN AND VEGETARIAN PROTEIN POWER

Before you freak out over our love of animals, let us say that we are aware that you *can* get complete proteins by combining grains and beans. You still won't be able to completely make up for the boost in testosterone created by animal protein, but we realize that some of you won't eat animals for moral reasons. Many vegan-friendly sources can help you reach your protein goals, but from our experience it's harder without the help of meat.

Then again, that's why protein powders exist. And if you're vegetarian, then you can enjoy eggs. And the pescatarians can have fish. So we have nothing against this population, and vegetarians and vegans will definitely benefit from our diet; however, we will not be specifically providing a vegetarian diet. Sorry. It's not personal. Everything we've seen and all the science we've read indicate that vegetarianism—while healthy—will not optimize your hormones. And that's our primary goal.

THE WORLD'S BEST MEAT

As two of the world's foremost carnivores, we've done our fair share of eating protein. And there are few things we enjoy more than cooking up our own grass-fed, organic steaks. While organic foods can be overrated, that is not the case with meats and fresh produce. The best meat we have found is provided by U.S. Wellness Meats. We ordered cases of meat during the writing process, and this protein fueled not only our bodies but also our minds. Trust us on this one: their customer service is top-notch, and the only things better are the taste, flavor, and variety. If you're looking for something a little more rare (pun intended), check out Exotic Meats USA—they have some really interesting choices, ranging from crocodile to black bear. For our favorite cuts of meat, visit www.engineeringthealpha.com.

■ *HOW MUCH PROTEIN DO I NEED?*

One of the most frequently asked questions about protein is, how much?

The interesting thing about that question is that it really encompasses two completely separate and diametrically opposed viewpoints. The first is minimalist: How much protein do I need to eat? Or, more succinctly, what is the minimal effective dose? Then, there is the maximalist: How much protein can I eat? Which really means, how much protein can I eat before it becomes either ineffective or dangerous?*

In order to best answer these questions, we'll look at this from the perspectives that matter most: fat loss and muscle gain. In both of these cases, the answer is a lot lower than you'd expect.

Fat Loss

For fat loss, you can really get away with as little as 0.5 grams per pound of LBM—which for most people will be anywhere between 60 and 90 grams of protein. A remarkably low number, compared to what you hear from most fitness pros.

Now, as we said, this is a minimalist approach . . . and so 0.5 grams per pound of LBM should be enough to help you hang on to all your lean mass, drop fat, and keep energy levels up. Having said that, it's arguable that a slightly higher intake of protein would allow you to

---

* *If you really want to understand the truth about how much protein you do (or don't!) need, pick up the book* How Much Protein? *by Brad Pilon.*

lose fat a little faster because of the thermic effect of food. Protein is very metabolic, meaning that up to 30 percent of the calories are burned during the digestion process. Another thing to consider is satiety. Higher protein consumption leads to greater satiety after eating, and so you'd be less hungry, and that makes it a lot easier to be compliant with your eating plan.

Muscle Gain

A minimalist approach to protein for muscle gain is really interesting; again, you actually need a lot less protein than you'd imagine.

In fact, in most cases, you could get away with 0.5 grams to 1 gram per pound of LBM. That's right—assuming you are consuming adequate calories, there is some research to illustrate that, provided you're getting all essential amino acids, you can gain muscle with as little as 0.5 grams per pound of LBM, according to The International Society of Sports Nutrition.

If this seems extremely low, it's because it is. Nevertheless, the research illustrates that it's accurate, and we've seen a few people thrive on this.

HOW TO EAT MORE PROTEIN WHEN LOSING FAT

If you're like us, you want to find out how to squeeze in as much protein as possible. We have experimented quite a lot with low-carb and high-protein diets, and we find that the more intense your weight training is, the more protein you can ingest and utilize before you have to worry much about gluconeogenesis. This is, very probably, due to the fact that intense weight training increases levels of testosterone, which in turn increases the rate of protein synthesis and nitrogen retention.

Therefore, we would argue that even on a low-carb diet, if you're training intensely and as long as calories are still low enough to allow for fat loss, you can do exceedingly well setting protein intake at around 1 gram per pound of LBM as a jumping-off point. All of that, again, applies primarily to low-carb diets where insulin control is the primary goal.

Most of our clients use some form of carb cycling, which we'll explain in part 3, and in this case protein intake fluctuates along with carbohydrate intake. In that situation, we'll often go as high as 1.25 grams of protein per pound of LBM, which we find allows for satiety without any detrimental effect on the rate of fat loss.

That said, we don't really care for the minimalist approach, mainly because if we take in the minimal amount of protein and still look to have adequate calories . . . well, those calories have to come from somewhere, and your choices are carbs and fat. We don't see the need to sacrifice convenience and satiety simply to keep protein as low as possible.

Which is why we prefer a maximalist approach to protein. This is about eating as much protein as you can get away with eating before it becomes either counterproductive relative to your goals or unhealthy.

For the purposes of fat loss, if you're taking in too much protein—upward of 2 grams per pound of body weight—the amino acids will be broken down into glucose or substances that react very much like sugar. Put simply: protein becomes carbs. (Well, sort of. But you get the idea.)

Which means this: if you are on a diet that depends on insulin control, it is detrimental to overeat protein. Some studies have shown that gluconeogenesis can occur with as little as 0.8 grams of protein per pound of LBM. But as a general rule (and one that's very easy to calculate), we recommend starting at 1 gram per pound of LBM and playing around from there.

HIGH PROTEIN AND KIDNEY PROBLEMS: MORE BULLSHIT

Some "experts" would like to have you believe that eating lots of protein will cause all sorts of problems, ranging from kidney stones and gallstones to extra arms growing out of your face.

For most people, this is not a concern—or rather, it is a moot point. We say this because there's no research showing any relationship between eating lots of protein and developing kidney problems. In fact, a study in the *Journal of Strength and Conditioning Research* tested up to 400 grams of protein per day without any negative consequences.

Now, if you have a preexisting kidney problem, it's possible that a higher protein diet could be hard on your body. But if you have a kidney problem, you should be talking to your doctor about your diet anyway. If you're healthy, you are clear to eat protein and not worry about any health problems. Because there are none. But remember, protein still contains calories. So if you eat tons of protein, you will eventually gain weight. The laws of thermogenesis do not bend for protein, even if it is delicious.

Again, the exact formulas are coming soon. We just don't want to worry about explaining once we get to the program. By that time, we hope you can dig in, get it, and begin your transformation.

For those of you looking to gain muscle and eat tons of protein, set your intake at about 1.5 grams per pound of your desired LBM, which means that if you currently have 160 pounds of lean mass and you'd like to gain 10 pounds of muscle, just multiply 170 by 1.5 and arrive at 255 grams of protein. Move up from there as needed or desired.

Of course, high protein intake can help with muscle; after all, isn't it true that eating more protein can lead to a more anabolic environment in your body? Well, that's certainly what the muscle magazines would have you believe. And, to be fair, it is true—to a point.

However, it is very important to note that, once again, we're dealing with diminishing returns. Which means that you will not gain more muscle eating 400 grams of protein per day than you will eating 300 grams of protein per day.

CHAPTER 7

The End of Dieting

WHY INTERMITTENT FASTING WILL CHANGE YOUR BODY AND YOUR LIFE

"What some call health, if purchased by perpetual anxiety about diet, isn't much better than tedious disease."

—ALEXANDER POPE

f you're like us, then you probably love the title of this chapter. Well, that's good, because it might be the most powerful, controversial, and *accurate* title in the book. We are going to put an end to dieting.

Sound far-fetched? Don't worry, we like it when people doubt us. But before we get into why *not dieting* is going to lead to the fastest fat loss you've ever had, let's create context. Here's how most fitness and nutrition experts like to handle the subject of what you eat:

It's not a diet, it's a lifestyle.

Diet is a four-letter word.

Organic diets are the only healthy diets.

Shop the perimeter and eat more real food.

If it's Paleo, it's not good.

Okay, maybe we made that last one up.

Let's clear something up fast: everyone has a diet. A diet, by definition, is what you eat. So unless you're starving and never eating, then you have a diet. What people are really talking about is diet*ing*—the idea of altering what you eat to follow a few simple, or not-so-simple, rules designed to help you be healthier, lose weight, or just not have terrible allergic reactions to some dangerous foods.

The problem with dieting—well, one of the many problems—is that men don't respond to food like women do. After training thousands of clients, a few things are exceedingly clear to us: men aren't successful when they subsist solely on frozen entrees; they don't adapt to vague recommendations like "eat low carbs." Instead they want specific guidelines; and they most certainly don't avoid pleasures like pizza, beer, and burgers. Once you acknowledge these things, it's pretty hard to imagine a "diet" on which men can be successful—unless you look at the science.

Conventional dieting wisdom posits that you need to change your lifestyle, that you need to eat prepackaged meals to fit your busy lifestyle, and that you need to avoid pizza and burgers. Conventional dieting wisdom says that you're not *supposed* to be able to eat those unhealthy foods and still lose fat each week.

But the science of dieting has made the concept of food restriction almost obsolete—only few people have paid attention enough to realize how much flexibility actually exists.

Forget about good foods versus bad foods; that argument no longer matters. Read that again: from a body composition standpoint,* *it doesn't matter* if you eat dry grilled chicken or a juicy burger; it doesn't matter if you choke down cottage cheese or pound some Ben & Jerry's. Whatever you're thinking, it doesn't matter.

All that matters . . . is timing and calories.

The nature of your endocrine system is incredibly complicated—but once you understand it, eating becomes easier than ever. Manipulate the times that you eat and you can eat and drink whatever you want and still look like a Greek god.

How? It's all locked in the secrets of the hormones leptin and ghrelin (see chapter 5 for a reminder) and the anabolic nature of the foods you eat.

Normally, when people go on a diet, they don't eat *as much* bad stuff . . . but they still eat it pretty consistently. They're making progress, but they're not there yet. It's an undergraduate approach to eating: one foot in, one foot out. While this approach can work, as you're (hopefully) reducing calories, it's incredibly limited. In fact, it's one of the least effective approaches for fat loss (trumped only in inefficacy by nonsense like cabbage soup and cayenne pepper).

Here's why: when you diet hard and drop calories significantly for a few days, leptin begins to drop. Again, leptin is a master hormone, and it's partly responsible for regulating

---

* This means that in terms of losing fat and gaining muscle, the foods are irrelevant; however, from a health perspective, that isn't necessarily the case. So in the words of Howard Stern's father, "Don't be an idiot, you moron." Eat your favorite foods, but be sure to eat some veggies every once in a while, mmmkay?

your thyroid. And your thyroid is integral to your ability to lose weight. So when your leptin levels drop, so too do thyroid hormones T3 and T4. When this happens, your metabolism slows down dramatically, and you lose *less* weight.

Think about that for a minute—you eat less and your weight loss slows down. That hardly seems fair. But that's what happens when your hormones work against you. Thankfully, there's a way to make them work *for* you.

Remember, leptin levels have a direct relationship with caloric intake. This means that just as leptin levels fall when you take in fewer calories, they rise when you take in more calories—and they rise a lot when you take in a ton of calories all at once. And, with very few exceptions, it *doesn't* matter where those calories come from.

So to prevent fat-loss stagnation and the dreaded weight-loss plateau, we need to make sure that we consistently spike your leptin levels when it drops too low. The way to do this is so awesome that it's hard to believe: you spend an entire day once per week eating whatever you want. Your nutritionist might call it a strategic overfeed 'cause they like to act all fancy, but colloquially, this is known as a cheat day.

The cheat—er, strategic overfeed—bumps your leptin levels up, allowing you to lose fat again. This means that you'll actually lose fat faster than if you had no cheat day at all. So even though you take in a ton of calories, the hormonal impact from the cheat offsets what you eat in a way that has a much greater benefit than if you avoided the splurge altogether.

And when we say a ton of calories, we mean men should be eating what they want. Enjoy pizza and burgers. Then grab dessert. Go crazy because it's an essential part of the plan. And it'll make any of the normal hardships of dieting nonexistent.

All told, in a very real sense, it's better to eat this stuff all at once in a single day than to have a little bit every day. We know, we know—that sounds crazy. It runs counter to all conventional nutritional wisdom. Well, sorry it doesn't make sense, but we didn't invent the science—we just report it and make it work.

But this dream situation only works with a specific approach: intermittent fasting.

WHAT IS INTERMITTENT FASTING?

The most accurate definition is the simplest one: intermittent fasting is merely alternating intervals of not eating (fasting) with times when you are allowed to eat.

We'll admit that most people usually freak out over this concept.

What? No eating? But what about starvation mode? What about feeding my metabolism? What about going into a severe catabolism so great that I have no energy and I can't build muscle?

By now, we hope we've convinced you—with science and real life results—that those are just myths. That line of thinking is why so many people struggle to look and feel better. This is about remembering that you need to step outside of the Ordinary World in order to create an unreal life.

But when you take a closer look at the reality of intermittent fasting, you quickly realize that the concept isn't crazy or uncommon. In fact, everyone practices a variation of intermittent fasting each day. When you sleep, you fast. When you awake, you eat. That's intermittent fasting. Not so bad, right?

And it also happens during your typical workday. When you're stuck in meetings all day and don't have a meal for five hours, that's technically fasting. The only difference is that you aren't on a structured timetable of meals in which the window of fasting is constant, so rather than fasting intermittently, you're fasting *haphazardly*—and there's no benefit.

All we're going to do is teach you how to ever so slightly expand your fasting window so you can experience the benefits of burning more fat, building more muscle, improving aging, boosting your sex drive, fighting off disease, looking more attractive, and strengthening your overall health. Oh yeah, and when you fast intermittently, you have rules, but *you* are in control.

It's a simplified approach. And while it's detailed and calculated, everything revolves around one easy-to-follow principle: eat by your clock. You set the hours that you eat. And then you have enhanced food freedom unlike any program you've ever tried before.

There are several variations of intermittent fasting, and we're going to show you how to integrate each one during the four phases of the program for the best results. The fasting period you'll use can range anywhere from sixteen hours all the way up to thirty-six hours (with several stops in between), and each of those plans has specific benefits. In the diet part of the program, we'll show you exactly when you need to apply each form of fasting and make it simple for you to make this new form of eating feel effortless.

INTERMITTENT FASTING IS THE ANSWER

If intermittent fasting is the answer, you're probably wondering about the question. It's really the only question any guy wants to ask when it comes to dieting: Is there an eating approach that puts me in control and actually works?

If you look at all the research, compare the high-fat diets to low-fat, the high-carb programs to low-carb, and the protein to more-protein (because every diet needs protein), you discover something that would surprise most people. Many diets work. There is no magic bullet. There is no "killer" food that ruins your eating plan. That's just not how our bodies work. But what causes diets to fail are psychological and social limitations that men don't deal with—no booze, no late-night eating, or no burgers. You need something with rules that work but also flexibility that allows you to have a life you can enjoy—and a body you can enjoy looking at.

On the most basic level, only two things matter: the calories you eat and taking in some balance of macronutrients—proteins, carbs, and fats. The manipulation of those macronutrients and calories on a daily, weekly, or monthly basis is the special sauce that allows for progress. In our program sometimes you'll find that you'll eat fewer carbs. Other times it'll be fat. And in other situations you will need *more* protein . . . and carbs . . . and fats to reach your goals.

So if all foods are fair game and eating some bad foods is actually okay, then why do so many people struggle with their diet?

It's because the system of eating is broken. It's based on mistruths, mistakes, and dogma. People are taught that eating can only be done *one* way, and their indoctrination creates a system in which their body always wants and expects food. They burn less fat because they spend too much time eating. And they struggle with binges because they're told to resist the foods they love—which of course only results in them eating *more* of those foods than they would otherwise.

This is why intermittent fasting is so successful. It eliminates all the problems that cause you to fail. We'll walk you through the different forms of intermittent fasting soon, but before we do, it's important that you understand why it works and why it's not only the most flexible plan you could find—but also much healthier than most believe.

DIET FIX #1: MORE FLEXIBILITY TO CHOOSE WHEN YOU EAT

People's first reaction whenever we bring up intermittent fasting is always the same: don't we *need* breakfast?

Most people on an intermittent fasting plan forego eating during traditional breakfast time; instead of eating first thing in the morning, they have their first meal in the afternoon. (Although as you'll see, you can still follow an intermittent fasting schedule and eat early in the morning.) This advice is exactly the opposite guidance bestowed by every authority from registered dietitians to MDs.

For years, we've been told that breakfast is the most important meal of the day. In fact, physicians are notorious for scolding patients who skip breakfast—particularly people who are embarking on a plan to lose weight.

There *is* some credence here, by the way: a study conducted by researchers at Virginia Commonwealth University in 2008 showed that participants who ate a calorically dense breakfast lost more weight than those who didn't. The espoused theory was that the higher caloric intake early in the day led people to snack less often throughout the day and lowered caloric intake overall. There are also some epidemiological studies that show a connection between skipping breakfast and higher body weight.

However, the crux of the breakfast study is ultimately that a larger breakfast leads to lower overall caloric intake. That is, the argument for a larger breakfast ultimately boils down to energy balance; if that study is reliant on the position that weight loss comes down to calories in versus calories out, then the makeup of the food shouldn't matter. If we've learned anything from Mark Haub's Twinkie Diet, it's that you can eat garbage and lose weight; so clearly, something else is going on.

The only real argument the breakfast crowd has is insulin sensitivity. As you've learned by now, the more sensitive your body is to insulin, the more likely you are to lose fat and gain muscle. Increasing insulin sensitivity almost always leads to more efficient dieting.

The pro-breakfast folks declare that because insulin sensitivity is higher in the morning, eating a carbohydrate-rich meal early in the day is the greatest opportunity to take in a large amount of energy without the danger of weight gain.

There's only one tiny problem with that theory: insulin sensitivity is *not* higher in particular hours of the morning. It's higher after a minimum of eight hours of *fasting*. It just so happens that you fast when you sleep, so the information is misleading. More specifically, insulin sensitivity is higher when your glycogen levels (the energy stores in your body) are depleted, like after your sleeping fast.

Intermittent fasting takes that a step farther and turns your body into a fat-burning, muscle-building machine. You see, if you skip breakfast and extend the fasting period beyond the typical eight to ten hours, you increase insulin even more.

Does this make a difference? You bet it does—both internally, in terms of the efficiency with which your body functions, *and* externally, with how you look.

But that's just the beginning. Insulin sensitivity is also increased after you exercise (due to further glycogen depletion), in which case if you can train in your fasted state in the morning and then eat, you have set your body up to maximize fat burning in the morning. What's more, you turn *all* your post-workout meals—so everything you eat the rest of the day—into super fuel that will have you looking leaner and more muscular, and feeling more satisfied and energized than ever before.

In the end, there is no science that supports the idea—from a direct comparison—that eating breakfast is better than not eating breakfast. Some people might have a psychological dependence or belief that it's what they need, or they could have a habit of binging when they are hungry. But from a physiological perspective, as in how your body actually reacts to breakfast, there's nothing special about eating early in the morning. In fact, forcing yourself to eat at a particular time, or a prescribed number of times, is just as big of a problem as saying you need breakfast.

DIET FIX #2: YOU CHOOSE HOW OFTEN YOU EAT

The reason why so many people hate dieting is that there's too much confusion about what you can and can't eat. Calorie-restrictive plans like Weight Watchers certainly don't agree with plans like the Atkins diet, the first iteration of which allowed dieters to eat all they wanted as long as they kept carbs low. As we've already mentioned, this confusion goes out the window with intermittent fasting, as it offers much more freedom to eat foods that you enjoy.

Despite the incredibly disparate nature of most diets, the one thing that has been consistently suggested in most books published over the past twenty years is the frequency of meals.

If you've read a diet book, seen a nutritionist, or hired a personal trainer at any point during that time, you've probably been told that in order to lose weight, you need to eat five to six small meals per day.*

This style of eating, commonly referred to as the frequent feeding model, is popular with everyone from dietitians to bodybuilders and has been repeated so often for so long that it's generally taken as fact.

But it's not.

The reputed benefits of eating frequent, small meals have never been scientifically validated, although there have been studies that have tried. The theory suggests that since eating increases your metabolic rate, the more often you eat, the more your metabolic rate will be elevated. But this has never been conclusively shown.

That part is actually true, by the way. Every time you put food in your mouth, you burn calories. When you eat, your inner machinery needs to work hard to break down the food you eat; the breakdown and conversion of food into energy *requires* some energy itself, and some is used to help you walk, think, breathe, build muscle, lose fat, and even sleep. Some.

And the rest? Well, the leftovers require energy to be transported as adipose tissue—the bad stuff that gives you love handles—or broken down and passed through your digestive tract.

Going a bit farther, we know that the amount of energy you burn depends on the food you eat. This is known as the thermic effect of food. Of all the foods you eat, protein is the most metabolically expensive—it costs more energy to break down, digest, and put to use than either carbohydrates or fat. Up to 30 percent of the calories you eat from protein are burned during the digestion and processing of those foods.

That's one of the main reasons why diets with protein are so great; the more protein you eat, the more calories you burn. Carbohydrates are less metabolically active (about 6 to 8 percent burned), and fats are the least metabolically active (about 4 percent burned) despite being the highest in calories and great for your testosterone levels.

---

* You may have also heard this recommendation phrased as "3 meals and 3 snacks."

Now, here's where things got muddy for a while: it was posited that if eating requires energy, then eating more frequently would require energy more frequently—and that a net effect would be to require more energy. That's how the multiple-meals-per-day movement started. Makes sense from a logical perspective, but it's completely based on pseudoscience and assumptions. Shockingly, no one questioned this for decades.

The *reality* is that your body doesn't care about how many meals you eat. Read that again and write it down because it might be the biggest change that improves your new approach to food. You can choose how often you want to eat every day.

The thermic effect of food is directly proportional to caloric intake, and if caloric intake is the same at the end of the day, there will be no metabolic difference between eating six meals or three.

This fact is so blatantly true that Canadian researchers wrote a published study that was literally titled: "Increased Meal Frequency Does Not Promote Greater Weight Loss in Subjects Who Were Prescribed an 8-Week Equi-Energetic Energy-Restricted Diet." (We think they were trying to make the point clear.) In fact, as long as the total calories are the same, you can eat ten meals or one meal and you'll still get the same metabolic effect.

The best approach to your diet is the one that is sustainable for you and fits your lifestyle. With regard to energy balance and thermic effect of food, you can really eat as many meals—or as few—as you want. Your body primarily functions based on how much you eat, the composition of what you eat, and the sources of food you select. Yes, there are strategies that you should follow—such as eating more carbs late at night. But whether you split those carbs into one big meal or three nightly snacks is your choice.

There are reasons why eating less frequently could be a better choice for you and your body. Researchers at the University of Kansas Medical Center found that eating more frequently is less beneficial from the perspective of satiety, or feeling full. Which means that the more often you eat, the more likely you are to be hungry—leading to higher caloric intake and eventual weight gain. In other words, whether you realize it or not, when you eat more often, you're more likely to eat more food. When you eat less frequently, you can eat larger meals and feel more satisfied, and you're less likely to take in more calories.

This also makes sense if you're following an intermittent fasting routine to limit the number of hours you eat during the day. If you condense the amount of time you allow yourself to eat into a small window of four to eight hours, having more than two to three meals becomes impractical at best and impossible at worst. That's why most of our clients prefer to have just two to three meals, and they find that this works perfectly with their schedule and lifestyle. If more meals are needed, that's fine too—as long as it works within the intermittent fasting schedule and the eating window (eight to ten hours, on most days) that you create.

Whatever you choose, these two fixes offer you more control than other dieting methods do, and their lack of control is one of the most common reasons why people quit eating plans.

THE HEALTHIEST, MOST SCIENTIFICALLY SUPPORTED DIET EVER CREATED

The most obvious reasons to follow an intermittent fasting protocol is that there really aren't any downsides and it's the only eating strategy to help optimize hormones, according to what we've found within scientific literature. For starters, there's the improved insulin sensitivity that comes with fasting, especially when paired with the exercises in part 3. Fasting also increases the secretion of GH, offsets cortisol production, helps control leptin and ghrelin levels to keep you satisfied, and even facilitates a healthier environment for testosterone production. It's a hormone optimization cocktail that depends on only one action—setting a window of time for when you eat. And that window can shift based on the day and your schedule.

We'll be the first to admit that intermittent fasting isn't for everyone. Some people might try it and not like the approach. But for health benefits and ease of application, you won't find many dieting strategies with fewer rules. As you'll discover, after the initial phase, you're able to eat carbs, fats, proteins, and even dessert. You can eat breakfast—or skip it. You can drink alcohol—with the right approach—and you are even required to eat dessert on cheat days. All of the other dietary facts that are supported by science remain consistent with intermittent fasting. All that changes is that you choose an eating "window" that works best for your schedule, and simply shrink the number of hours that you eat. It's an adjustment, but one with many benefits and something you should try before you assume it's not going to work for you.

We realize that you might have some reservations. For most people, the main reservation is the fear of going into starvation mode or the idea that not eating for long periods of time is unhealthy. But we can assure you that you won't starve by going twelve hours, sixteen hours, or even thirty-six hours without food. The biggest blocks during the fasts will be mental. And we'll provide you with tricks and techniques to go longer periods without food, making your hunger pangs a thing of the past.

In the end, we just want people to look good, feel great, and live healthier lives. And that's what intermittent fasting offers. For people looking to drop weight, intermittent fasting can help people reduce food intake by 30 percent without increasing hunger. And because you're eating smaller amounts and less frequently, your body can look elsewhere in your body for energy, which encourages cellular repair. That is, a cell will turn to its own damaged proteins for energy. While that cycle would be bad in the long term, keep in mind you're only fasting for brief periods; when you eat again your body will be rejuvenated. All told, this phenomenon—which, again, stems from caloric restriction—can generally help prevent both disease and age.

We've already provided plenty of evidence of these health benefits. But to further deliver the point, researchers at the University of Utah found that people who fasted just *one day* per month were 40 percent less likely to suffer from clogged arteries. In the survey-based study, more than five hundred people had their regular habits assessed. These habits covered eating schedules, including fasting; choice to smoke or not; and consumption of or abstinence from caffeine or alcohol. And only one trait—fasting—was correlated with lower rates of heart disease. Even when adjusted for age, weight, cholesterol, diabetes, or high blood pressure, the difference between fasters and non-fasters still remained.

THE EASY GUIDE TO INTERMITTENT FASTING

We just offered a lot of information on why intermittent fasting is an incredibly effective way to eat and has more health benefits than any other diet plan. Quite simply, it seems as if we were designed to eat this way. And while it might be hard to believe, your body will adapt in less than a week, and the hunger pangs that you used to experience will disappear and be replaced with freedom and control.

But just in case you're feeling a little confused, these are the only rules:

1. Fast: Go without eating for a period of time. Most days, this will just be sixteen hours.

2. Eat: Select an eight-hour window—*any* eight-hour window—and use that as your eating time. You could start eating at 9:30 A.M. and then have your dinner at 5:30 P.M. For us, that means we start eating at two P.M. and end at ten P.M.

3. Be flexible: If you want to eat at ten A.M. one day or have a business breakfast planned, go for it. Ideally you'd just eat from ten A.M. to six P.M. Or if you don't want to start eating until four P.M., do that.

The best part about intermittent fasting is that it's designed to work for you. The restrictions are only related to overcoming your mental blocks and learning to control your hunger, which will become invaluable skills once you learn that your symptoms of hunger are more because of the eating schedule you've created than actually needing food.

Put it all together, and you start to see that intermittent fasting is not only misunderstood but is also the best plan for any type of person. When combined with exercise, it creates an optimal hormonal environment that will produce even greater results. And even if you choose *not* to exercise (although it's not what we'd recommend), intermittent fasting has been proven to be an effective weight-loss technique and a strategy that can mimic many of the health benefits of exercise, including fighting disease and improving longevity. For those who are active—as we recommend—intermittent fasting will enhance everything you do in the gym.

We know that letting go of your previously held beliefs can be difficult. And we acknowledge that for some people, it can take seven to ten days to adjust to an intermittent fasting schedule. But once you find a pattern that works for your lifestyle, you'll see that you'll never have to search for another diet again.

PART 3
ENGINEERING THE ALPHA

"FROM THE ASHES A FIRE SHALL BE WOKEN,
A LIGHT FROM THE SHADOWS SHALL SPRING;
RENEWED SHALL BE BLADE THAT WAS BROKEN,
THE CROWNLESS AGAIN SHALL BE KING."
—J. R. R. TOLKIEN, *THE FELLOWSHIP OF THE RING*

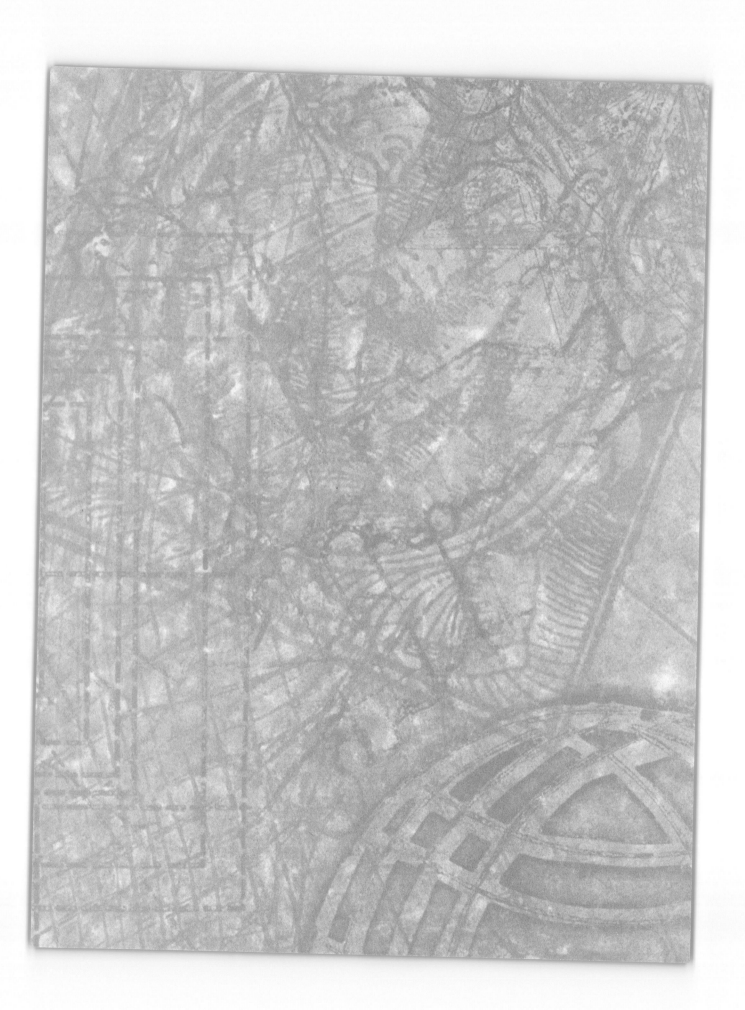

CHAPTER 8

The Road to Alpha Status

EATING, TRAINING, AND BUILDING THE BODY OF A GOD

*"I've missed more than 9000 shots in my career. I've lost almost 300 games;
26 times, I've been trusted to take the game winning shot and missed.
I've failed over and over and over again in my life. And that is why I succeed."*

—MICHAEL JORDAN

The best thing that ever happened to you was failure. This isn't another one of our jokes. This is real. Although frustrating, it's good that you've struggled in your goal to get the body you want, have been pissed off by bad diets, and might genuinely consider this your last-ditch effort to see if exercise really works.

We're okay with that. It's not that we want you to struggle, suffer, and become cynical. And while we certainly feel bad for those people who have been plagued by decades of frustration (you younger readers have trodden through less crap), we do know that these struggles were essential if you truly are to achieve an unreal life and an awesome body. That's because it's a necessary part of your journey and may be the most integral part to achieving Apotheosis.

The sixth stage of the Hero's Journey is the Road of Trials. One could argue that this is the most important phase because it is here that you will receive the knowledge and experience necessary to reach your ultimate goals. It's the process of earning your stripes, proving your keep, and being able to learn by doing—and occasionally failing—that has the most value. And now that you've spent time learning why everything works, now you can begin to take action.

As a phase, the Road of Trials serves as a series of tests that the hero must face to prepare him for the final challenge. But it's not all about beating the game or saving the princess—as we'll cover soon, the tests are a necessary step in the hero's development, preparing him for life after the challenge. The exposure to the tests—and both succeeding and failing—will teach him about the world and himself. The successes will allow him to keep moving forward on his journey. But the failures specifically are what will instruct him of his flaws, make him aware of his weaknesses, and spark a deeper drive to succeed.

FINDING THE EYE OF THE TIGER

Your tests started before you picked up this book. While not directly in order of the Hero's Journey, all those frustrations led you here. And it's a good thing you're here now because what you'll find in this section and beyond will lead to dramatic changes you wouldn't find unless you were placed in this situation. So if you never struggled, you'd never be able to open your eyes to what is really possible. And that's why your prior failures will ultimately be the spark that triggered your future success.

This concept is a mainstay of nearly every great story. Whether it's played out on a screen, on a page, or even in a video game. Looking at ancient mythology, Odysseus had to go through ten years of hell and endless obstacles to reach his final destination. King Arthur had to repeatedly overcome obstacles in his ascent to royalty and then in the quest of the Holy Grail. Even Link from *The Legend of Zelda* was constantly fighting increasingly difficult challenges to save Princess Zelda and her kingdom.

We could also look at sports and movies, but in the interest of brevity, we'll look at the best of both and examine sports movies, in particular the *Rocky* films. Choose any of those movies and you'll find instances of the Road of Trials. But maybe the most prominent is *Rocky III*. (It's also the first time in the series that Sly really gets shredded for his role—and it marks the birth of the "Eye of the Tiger.")

In this film, the movie opens with Rocky destroying everyone he fights. Only it turns out that these were handpicked opponents who wouldn't really challenge the aging fighter. In many ways, this opening holds the most importance for you.

In life, we like to find the opponents we *know* we can beat. Success is a drug. And we've mentioned many times that creating success is the key to experiencing more success. But there's a caveat. Success only has value if it's earned. That process of overcoming an obstacle or becoming better at a process is what gives you real confidence—not a façade of machismo—that allows you to control your universe. Don't settle for the easy path just because it's easy. Don't be afraid of failure. Because even if you fail, it can lead to something so much greater.

That's what happened to Rocky. Once he took on a real challenge—"Clubber" Lang—he was easily defeated.*

This was the road Rocky needed to take to become a real champion. He had to find something that created fear. And for him—that was the fear of losing. This allowed him to start training with Apollo, get back that eye of the tiger, get in ridiculous shape, and box like a fucking boss.

It was the failure—and the fear—that made him better. And it's what will make you better too.

EMBRACING YOUR REALITY: BE THE UNDERDOG

The Road of Trials is the reason why we like underdog stories. It resonates on a deep psychological level. We like to see a group of ragtag kids defeat the bad guy because we like to see development. It's inspirational. We love the process of taking the impossible and watching it become reality. But before reaching success, we have to deal with many struggles. And along the way, the obstacles become more difficult, thus preparing the underdog for success.

This same concept is played out in every aspect of life. To win the Super Bowl, you have to play well in the regular season, defeat a bunch of difficult opponents in the play-offs, and then peak for one sixty-minute game on the biggest stage. In baseball, you start on home base—and even if you knock it out of the park, you still have to run the bases. In relationships, you don't marry the first person you meet. You learn something from each relationship that helps you find the one.

The same holds true with fitness. You don't start out bench-pressing 300 pounds. You have to set benchmarks. You have tests and a journey. If you start at 135, your first goal is hitting 225. Then you'll progress up to 250, then 275, and finally 300.

Our goal in this book is to ensure that you actually experience a Road of Trials so you can guarantee success. We don't want you to be frustrated, but much like video game developers, we've devised different phases that will help you prepare for your final battle—having a body that looks fucking amazing and living an unreal life. Those are big goals, which means you need big tests. This goes beyond giving you hard workouts. You need to earn your way to this existence. And by doing so, you'll not only experience success, but more importantly, you'll be the one in control of maintaining, sustaining, and continuing your progress so your unreal life becomes your reality—rather than a fleeting moment in time.

---

* Yes, we realize that Mickey was dying during the match. But let's be honest: Rocky wasn't beating Mr. T without some help.

ENGINEERING THE ALPHA

SUBJECT: *Mitch Hurn*

THE ORDINARY WORLD

When this all started I weighed 293 pounds. I had completed one of Roman's programs before, but then I fell back into back habits. After a terrible six months I gained a lot back. It was a frustrating experience and one that needed to change. I could either take a temporary approach, or go in with a new mind-set. I decided it was time to leave the old me, and my comfort zone.

ACCEPTING THE CALL

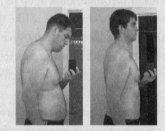
This time it was going to be different; I had a better plan than before, and higher drive to become the best version of myself. I wanted to be an Alpha. My personal goals were going to be difficult but attainable, and I went in with eyes wide open. I knew it was going to take a lot of hard work, new challenges, new eating strategies, and the drive to do that one last set or rep. I accepted a new approach to my health, and I believed in what I could become. I knew I was making progress when I was at the gym doing goblet squats and the weight I was using was higher than the amount of weight I have lost.

ALPHA STATUS

It's a whole new life for me. I feel better, look better, and have loads more energy than ever before and look forward to coming home at night and going to the gym. Other than marrying my wife, starting Roman's program has been the greatest decision of my life. I've already lost fifty pounds, lost five inches from my waist, and while I used to be an XXL, I can now fit into a large shirt.

When I started I had pain in my lower back and my knees would be screaming after the workouts. Now both areas are stronger than ever, and I no longer have pain. I can't express my thankfulness enough. I've already transformed so much, but I'm still excited to see how much more I can improve and what those changes will do for my life.

HIT THE ROAD: THE FOUR PHASES OF ENGINEERING THE BODY OF THE ALPHA

Your body transformation happens in four phases. Each phase has a distinct focus and scientific design that will solve all of the problems that typically hold you back, create plateaus, or just cause a lack of inspiring results. But before we give you the exact details, we want you to be prepared for what you're going to experience. Just as importantly, we want you to understand what you'll be doing and why you'll be doing it. You'll see why our approach is unique, and you'll understand the type of results you can expect to see.

PHASE I: PRIME

The Foundation: Building Your New Body

Chinese wise man Lao-Tsu said, "A journey of a thousand miles begins with a single step," the implication being that the first step is the hardest and most important. We certainly agree. Within the context of engineering the Alpha, the most important steps toward greatness occur in the beginning as well: heeding the Call to Adventure and Meeting the Mentor—all the things we've discussed so far are crucial to the success of this program.

But even within the workout and diet program itself, the first phase is also the most important. It sets the stage for everything else that will occur in the ensuing weeks and phases. Phase I is all about insulin. This hormone is a threshold guardian standing between you and the next phase of your development. Just as you have to pay Charon to ferry you across the River Styx, you must take control of insulin to take power over your body.

The Diet

The foundation of the first phase is an insulin reset. This is a strategic approach to your nutrition that will do exactly what the name implies—reset your insulin. And we mean that literally. Ultimately, the goal is to increase your insulin sensitivity, which is the first step to making your body better at building muscle and losing fat. And the intermittent fasting approach we use has been proven to speed up your metabolism and burn more fat, according to a study published in the *American Journal of Clinical Nutrition*. What is important about this study is that it was done in non-obese individuals. You see, most studies usually focus on the obese—people with a BMI upward of 30. While BMI is not the best indicator of a person's fitness level, it's pretty accurate for the sedentary, which is exactly the population that tends to be studied.

And while we've already seen research that shows intermittent fasting works for obese populations and sustains weight loss (an important point because most diets are not sustainable), this study showed that it worked for normal weight and healthy people too. This means that science supports the hypothesis that an insulin reset will burn fat for everyone.

We'll be honest: the amount of research on intermittent fasting in healthy populations is limited. And it's not because studies haven't confirmed our philosophy; it's because very few studies have analyzed the topic. You need to understand that getting funding for scientific research is extremely hard. And that's why lots of cool topics never have any research behind them. Trust us—we've been in the university environment and have gone through the frustrations ourselves. Getting funding is the worst part of a researcher's job. (That noise you hear, it's all the researchers reading this book simultaneously saying, "Mmmm hmmmmm.")

So given that reality, we decided to run our own scientific experiment. We tested the insulin reset on *all* kinds of people. Fat clients, thin clients, those who wanted to lose weight, and those who wanted to pack on muscle. In fact, we even tried the insulin reset on Arnold Schwarzenegger himself.

The results were undeniable. Two years of testing and thousands of subjects later, we had all the proof we needed.

It works.

By limiting your carbs—and timing them for the moments when you need them most—we retrain your body to manage the master hormone the right way. That is, there's a direct relationship between insulin management and nutrient uptake: the more insulin sensitive you are, the more nutrients (especially from carbs) will be directed into your muscle cells rather than your fat cells.

Inevitably, this is what will allow you to take in more carbs without becoming fat—and what will help turn cheat days into fat-destroying splurges.

During this initial phase, you'll be eating slightly below what is known as maintenance calories. Don't worry, once you see the menu of steak, bacon, and eggs, you'll realize that you'll be eating more than enough to be satisfied. The reason we're dropping your calories is to help burn off extra fat. Whereas most guys think they need to add muscle first and then cut fat, the best way to add more muscle is to start by dropping fat and improving insulin sensitivity. And that's exactly what you'll accomplish.

Just as important is what the introduction of intermittent fasting will do for your growth hormone (GH) levels. Before we even begin to focus on what training will do, simply adding intermittent fasting to your lifestyle can cause a *2,000 percent increase* in GH, according to research published by cardiologists at the Intermountain Heart Institute.

How can you get up to a 2,000 percent increase? Easily. Eat more before you go to sleep. A lot more. And then get at least six hours of rest. When you wake up, *don't* eat. Your GH peaks in the night and then shuts off the moment you have your morning eggs. Instead, drink some water, tea, or coffee, and push back breakfast a few hours. And just like that, your GH levels have surged and you've created a better environment for building muscle, melting fat, and fighting off aging. Not only is the burst more intense, but you'll also experience more frequent increases in GH throughout the day, which will keep the fat melting off your abs.

We've found that the insulin reset can be a difficult adjustment for some for about three to five days, as you adjust to a new style of eating. After that, you adjust and wonder why you ever ate any other way—your energy will be increased, your focus better, your stomach always satisfied, and your weight dropping. In fact, by now, you'll be in love with fasting and your body will be as insulin sensitive as possible without having to abstain from carbs for years. Again, this means that everything you eat is more likely to wind up packing mass on your arms instead of fat on your ass.

The Training

As with everything in this program, the diet is only half of the equation. Your first month of training (Phase I) is designed to improve your insulin sensitivity as well as start increasing production of testosterone and GH. We start with an intensive focus on fat loss, as that's the best and fastest way to reset your insulin. While the workouts are metabolic and crank up your ability to burn calories—both in and out of the gym—they are also designed to teach and reinforce the movement patterns that you need to master in order to get the most out of the program.

This is an important distinction between our approach and other fitness books. We want to mimic the approach you would receive if you worked with us one-on-one rather than just throw you into a program that expects you to automatically squat and deadlift like a pro. That's what frustrates us more than anything and why it's so hard for us to train in commercial gyms. No one teaches anymore. It's not your job to know how to exercise correctly; it's your job to be shown and to learn. The workouts in Phase I will give you the same benefits as very technical exercises without forcing you into mastery at such an early stage. Even if you're already a vet of the gym, this progression will make your body more efficient and will inevitably increase your strength gain and your fat loss. Just trust us on this. It's not as much one step back as it is three steps forward—without you even realizing it.

The Mind-Set

Phase I is also about getting your head right. This is arguably the hardest stage because we'll be introducing new strategies—like fasting—into your world. This is your trial by fire. This phase, while only the beginning, determines your worth and how suitable you are for the quest. Think of it like a knight's challenge or a test to become a Jedi. Like any threshold, this one is difficult to cross, but it prepares you for greater challenges. More importantly, once you get through this phase, your body will adjust and the entire process will become easier.

The adaptation curve is where most people quit and fail because it's their first step outside of their comfort zone and out of the Ordinary World. If you can hold tight, stay focused, and keep your eye on the prize, your body will adapt. And you will realize that you can get through anything else we throw at you. This applies to training and any other situation in life. Just like that, we will have created a structure of success, confidence, and happiness—and that cycle will be perpetuated throughout the process until you completely change your body and your mind-set.

This isn't meant to intimidate you. Instead, it's meant as motivation so you can rise up to the challenge. Because we'll be honest: the nature of this programming is such a drastic change from what most people prescribe that the result of Phase I is some pretty amazing progress. While we were testing this program on our clients, the average weight loss during Phase I was ten pounds. In fact, when Arnold Schwarzenegger* first tried the insulin reset, he lost four pounds in just two weeks. Not bad for a guy who's already in good shape.

In terms of sex drive, results are mixed. Some of our test subjects experience resurgence in their mojo, which we attribute to increased insulin sensitivity. Remember, insulin resistance inhibits blood flow and has been linked to erectile dysfunction. Admittedly, some people do experience a small dip in sex drive. This change is most likely due to a decrease in calories; thankfully, every single one of these clients reported a huge rebound effect in Phase II when testosterone becomes the greater focus.

In the end, Phase I is about big steps both mentally and physically. By the time you prepare for Phase II, you *will* be stronger and leaner, and feeling more capable and confident.

PHASE II: ADAPT

Unprecedented Territory: Reformulating the Rules of Fitness

Phase II is what we call Adapt—it's when you break out of the priming phase and cut yourself loose from the shackles of the insulin reset. Interestingly, what might have felt difficult in Phase I will now feel like the best diet you've ever tried.

But the progress isn't just on the diet side. After the first phase, you'll operate as an efficient machine in the gym. Some of the efficiency will result from familiarity. You'll now be well versed in the intensity and programming required to make real changes to your body. And we're not talking intensity in terms of workout duration, but in workout intent. You know how to focus and push yourself harder and more effectively than before. What's more, proper form will be ingrained into your very soul, and much like riding a

---

* Yeah, that's right: you're using the same diet we designed for the Terminator.

bike, there will be no going back. You know how your fingers can still execute the Konami Code,* even though you haven't picked up a Nintendo controller in years? That's how your form will be.

Your efficiency will be further buttressed by confidence. Most physiological changes are actually limited by psychological barriers. In ordinary life, we don't believe we can change, and then we find excuses to support why we failed. Many have said that the first person to bottle motivation will probably make a billion dollars. And while we haven't figured it out yet, we do know that confidence is just as good as the most potent bottled motivation. Because confidence is a drug—you will be hooked after the first phase and hungry for more.

The Diet

The most exciting part of Phase II occurs with your diet. And not just *kind of* exciting— we're talking the kind of excitement normally reserved for teenagers feeling their first boob. Yeah. What could rival pubescent over-the-clothes second base? Only one thing: cheat day, motherfucker.

All your hard work and strict abstinence and strategic timing of carbs in Phase I has paid off. Your body is not only primed to accept carbs, it's ready and waiting to make good use of them when strategically applied in larger quantities. During the cheat day, you will eat whatever you want. Anything at all. Pizza, burgers, wings, nachos. That's not to say that you can't keep it clean and have sweet potatoes, rice, oatmeal, and some lean meat.

Whatever Alpha wants, Alpha gets.

The Training

Phase II is also when things get serious in the gym. We're shifting from understanding intensity, work capacity, and mastering movement to manipulating other variables such as training density and frequency.

Density training will be employed to increase work capacity, enhance strength and endurance, and above all, increase your testosterone. Testosterone is the main focus because it's what will allow you to build more muscle and lose fat, but also because it's the under-

---

* Seriously, it pains us to have to explain this, but our editors insist. For those of you whose childhoods were so deprived that you didn't get to play games, the Konami Code is a cheat code that originated in the Konami game *Gradius,* giving the player extra lives and instant power-ups. The code is activated by entering ↑↑↓↓←→←→**BA** into the keypad and rose to prominence with the 1987 release of the Konami title *Contra*—during which the code granted the player thirty lives. It has since been used in hundreds of games. Easily the most well-known cheat code in the world, the Konami Code is part of geek culture. Out of interest, punk band the Ataris named a song "Up, Up, Down, Down, Left, Right, Left, Right, B, A, Start" after the Konami Code on their 2001 album, *End Is Forever;* ironically, the code never appeared on an Atari game.

lying problem that is restricting most men. Research shows that testosterone levels of the average man have dropped 30 percent during the past twenty years. It's time to change that. And using density training that emphasizes certain multi-muscle exercises (think: squats and deadlifts) is exactly the antidote for your lagging T levels.

Sex and Life

As your body changes, you'll also notice huge changes to your sex life. The increase in calories and carbs helps, but the hormonal surge of testosterone and GH (which exacerbates the effects of testosterone) will be responsible for your adolescent-like desire and drive.

Phase II is also where you'll experience the greatest increase in confidence. This is partially due to the undeniable and visible improvements in your physique and performance, and also to the more optimized hormonal environment. Not only are testosterone and GH now improved, but insulin will also be working in your favor instead of just being set to baseline levels of effectiveness.

As a result, you'll notice sometime around the middle of Phase II that you're thinking a bit differently. Brain function will increase, and you will actually get smarter. You probably won't notice this, but what you will notice is increased concentration and a general sense of focus, which will improve your productivity and effectiveness. You might also be faster to speak up and start to feel better in your relationship. Hell, maybe you'll just wear a tighter T-shirt. The point is that your entire worldview will begin to shift as a result of the increased confidence, and you'll have moved one step closer to realizing your potential and creating a happier, more satisfying universe.

PHASE III: SURGE

Breaking the Mold: The New Rules of Building Muscle

Any person who has ever been instructed about lifting weights understands that the process of building muscle must occur with some fat gain. In the bodybuilding world, this was known as a bulking phase. And it was a theory that actually seemed pretty sound: in order to build significant muscle, you need to eat more calories. It's true that those calories will help you become bigger, but inevitably some will spill over and turn into fat too.

As you know, we're not really fans of belly fat—or any body fat, for that matter. The only fat we like is that which comes on our steak. We just like adding muscle and eliminating fat. The key to making that happen is GH, which we'll trigger with some high-rep, high-intensity weight training. That's the big focus in Phase III—creating a surge in GH that helps you stay lean while adding size, and optimizing testosterone in a way that makes strength and muscle gains possible without adding fat.

The Diet

While lactic acid training and a boost in GH are certainly powerful, those alone wouldn't enable you to build muscle and stay lean at the same time. In order to accomplish this goal, we're going to strategically *increase* how much you eat on training days. That is, Phase III is the only stage where on every workout day you're eating significantly more than your maintenance level of calories. You'll lift hard and heavy, and then eat hard and heavy. These calories will be utilized toward growth. At the same time, on your non-exercise days you'll be eating significantly fewer calories.

This alternating-calorie approach has been shown by University of Virginia scientists to help maintain weight while gaining muscle and has been the secret to our success with all of our clients. That's because during the course of the week, your calories will still be at or below maintenance level. As we mentioned in Adapt, you'll be establishing your maintenance level of calories at the start of each phase, and Surge will be no different. But while in Surge, your overfeeding on your training days will help you build strength and muscle without fat.

The Training

Depending on how you view it, the Surge phase could either be the most fun part of the entire program or could intimidate you to the point of excitement. Every man needs to be able to rise to a challenge, and in order to promote more GH, you'll be pushing your body to the limit.

Each workout will utilize a total-body approach but will have an upper- or lower-body focus. For instance, you might start a workout with a multi-muscle lower-body movement like deadlifts. But we'll have you perform 20 reps of this movement and then follow with an entire upper-body workout of lactic acid–style training.

Lactic acid training is a difficult progression that increases the amount of time your muscles remain under tension. Time under tension is one of the most overlooked components of muscle growth, and it's important because this type of training has been shown to drastically increase output of GH. When combined, the concurrent *surge* in testosterone and GH makes every rep you perform, every set you complete, and all the food you eat prime for new growth. Research published in the *Journal of Applied Physiology* found that supplementation of testosterone and GH led to nearly three times the fat loss than achieved by taking either testosterone or GH individually. While these surges were due to supplementation, researchers speculated that elevating both levels naturally would have the same synergistic impact.

The day after lactic acid training, the order would be switched—starting with a compound upper-body lift (like a bench press or a push press) followed by lower-body lactic acid training. Don't worry about the exact details right now. Your easy-to-follow plan will be nicely laid out in chapter 11.

PHASE IV: COMPLETE
Living Like a Boss

Phase IV is the final stage. Here, you're able to combine all the elements of the first three phases into one meta approach. You can't typically do this in training because you have to build strategically in order for your body to reap the benefits of multiple techniques being utilized at the same time. This phase uses a mixed-methods approach to both training and diet that will change what is possible with your body.

Complete is a four-week phase. Here's what you can expect:

The Training

Weeks one and two are pure muscle building—you'll enjoy higher calories and carbs as well as a few meathead workouts mixed in with your density training. Because of the increases in strength and work capacity that were created in Phase II, you'll be able to make significant improvements much faster than normal. And that speaks to the overall design of this program. Every workout you perform is building toward a next step and something bigger. That's the science that we figured out so you wouldn't have to, and it's why our clients and the people who tested this program saw unprecedented and uncharacteristic results.

In week three, you'll throw your body a curveball by dropping calories and transitioning to a program based on pure strength. The goal here is to put the brakes on mass building in a way that prevents any fat gain while still cementing and fine-tuning your muscle gain with heavy lifting. Surprisingly, what you'll find is that even though your calories will be lower, your strength will *not* decrease. Much of this will be due to the peripheral benefits of intermittent fasting, but it's also because of the hormonal environment of improved insulin, GH, and testosterone. These hormones will sustain and bolster performance even in the absence of calories. And as your strength increases and your calories are lower, you'll be dropping fat at an accelerated rate.

In week four and beyond, we transition into a rotational program—one workout of various types each week. You'll still be eating just a tad below your maintenance level so you're able to stay lean, but you counterbalance that and keep leptin in check with a healthy dose of weekly epic cheat days.

Transformation

At the end of Phase III, your body will look radically different. You'll be leaner and bigger, but you'll also be harder and denser. These changes will be impossible not to notice. Just as beneficial, you'll *feel* different. You'll be mentally and emotionally centered, your increased confidence will have taken firm root, and you'll begin to explore new things with greater ease. You'll be more self-assured and self-reliant, so things won't distract you as much. And you'll have a sex drive that will reduce or completely eliminate one of the biggest stressors that all men experience—a lack of libido.

This is the reality of the more than three thousand men who have gone through this program. And now it's your turn.

CHAPTER 9

Phase I: Prime

ENGINEERING ENGAGED

"People do it every day. They talk to themselves. . . .
They see themselves as they'd like to be. They don't have the
courage you have, to just run with it."

—TYLER DURDEN IN *FIGHT CLUB*

ENGINEERING THE ALPHA: THE PROGRAM

The Engineering the Alpha training and nutrition program consists of four phases, each lasting three or four weeks. Every phase has a different purpose, and—with the exception of Phase IV—each will focus on helping you to optimize a specific hormone through diet and training. Phase IV is a bit more comprehensive, so rather than focusing on just a single hormone or modality, all of them are brought together in a cohesive fashion.

In order to accomplish this, each phase utilizes a different training style to elicit the desired effect. There are commonalities among all phases, of course. With regard to training, while each phase has you training in a different *way*, the exercises will be very similar. The reason for this is twofold. First, there are only so many amazing exercises; the fact is, while there are a thousand different pressing variations, you really only need three to five versions to build an incredible, well-balanced physique. The second point is that mastering a thousand pressing movements is impossible or, maybe more appropriately, counterproductive.

The truth is, in order to get the most out of any exercise, you have to be *good* at it. Or as we say in the industry, you have to have a high level of proficiency.* In other words, each set and rep you do is not only an end unto itself, but it's also—in a very real sense—practice for subsequent sets. By sticking with a core group of movements and branching out with slight variations of them, you'll be consistently improving rather than starting from scratch to learn new skills all the time.

A number of nutritional aspects will carry over from phase to phase as well. With the exception of your cheat days, you'll generally be eating a bit on the low-carb side (especially during Phase I). But as you'll come to discover, after the first two weeks, the definition of *low-carb* is actually many more carbs than most people think, which means you're not restricted as much as you'd expect on a typical low-carb plan.

There are two foundational nutritional principles of every phase of the diet: intermittent fasting and cycling.

Intermittent Fasting

During the program, you'll fast for anywhere from sixteen to thirty-six hours (that's not as bad as it sounds). How long each fast lasts will vary depending on which phase you're in, but some form of fasting will be utilized nearly every day. Not only does this allow for better results, but it also just makes life much more manageable without putting extra restrictions on what you eat and when you eat. Yes, there are rules, but you select the eating window, how many meals you eat during that window, and which foods you want to eat. Does this mean you can eat just crap? Of course not. But as you'll see from the Alpha-approved food list, not even a world-class chef would complain about the number of options available.

Cycling

In the context of dieting, *cycling* just means that you strategically alternate how much food you eat on a day-to-day basis. This means that on days you exercise, you eat more; on days you don't exercise, you eat less. Throughout the program you'll be cycling carbohydrates and total calories.

During various phases of the plan, you'll be eating up to three times as many carbs on workout days as you do on days you don't train. This is known as carb cycling, and has to

---

* You've no doubt caught on by now that we have a lot of very scientific terms to say very simple things; this is because half of the fitness industry is made up of smart guys trying to prove they're not meatheads, and the other half is meatheads trying to prove they're smart. This is one of the more hilarious things about the fitness industry. Others include fanaticism over diets, and a strange reticence of an entire industry to openly talk about sex despite the fact that all its advertising is based on wanting to look better naked. But we digress.

do with energy utilization and recovery. Put in the most succinct way possible, you need more energy on days you expend more energy.

Cycling calories and carbs is important for both hormonal optimization and body recomposition (shifting to a body with less fat and more muscle), but there's another advantage as well: researchers at Louisiana State University found in a 2005 study that calorie cycling prolongs your life. This conclusion was further supported by research conducted by the National Institutes of Health in 2008. This means calorie cycling has some pretty sweet benefits . . . if, you know, you like being alive longer.

GETTING STARTED WITH PRIME

Prime is intended to do just that: prime your body for everything to come. However, don't think of Prime as some sort of optional video game tutorial* that you can skip; this is arguably the most important phase. In fact, none of the other phases will be nearly as effective without it.

The diet, which will be explained soon, is the most important part of Phase I—nearly everyone coming into the program will have *some* level of insulin resistance (or insulin insensitivity). Because of this, the nutritional programming is designed to rapidly get your endocrine system back on track by immediately addressing insulin in a truly aggressive manner.

As for exercise, Phase I is set up for two very specific goals. For those relatively new to the gym or those who haven't trained in a while, the exercise setup of Phase I will have you seeing results fast. For everyone, it will set the foundation for the following three phases so you can experience exponential improvements. Even if you train regularly, learning the movements the way we want you to do them is going to take a little time. From a hormonal standpoint, Prime is geared toward improving insulin sensitivity, which will be accomplished through exercise as well as diet.

We'll talk about each of these benefits, but before we do, we just need to point out the obvious: synergy. By pairing a nutritional structure with a training approach, both of which are proven to improve insulin management, you increase the efficacy of both, allowing for not only rapid hormonal optimization but also rapid results in terms of fat loss and muscle gain.

---

* Those of you who have played first-person shooter games know what we're talking about here. For those who haven't, this is how it goes: Many games of that kind come with a tutorial chapter in the very beginning of the game; it serves no purpose other than to teach you the controls and familiarize you with the general mechanics of the game. There are no important plot points or development—just learning. This is boring and frustrating—and the opposite of what we want to accomplish with Phase I. Other games (the better ones) take a different approach and simply set up and pace the early part of the game in a way that teaches you the mechanics and allows you to develop your skills within the context of the story. This is what we want to accomplish for Phase I—we want you to build your skill set, certainly, but we want you to make actual progress while you do it. And you will.

Training Program

Phase I will be comprised of what is known as metabolic resistance training. This style of training uses resistance (either weights or your own body weight) in a fast-paced, circuit-style workout; circuits are executed with very little rest between exercises and are arranged in a noncompeting fashion. This means that you'll never work the same muscle in two consecutive exercises; rather, the exercise order alternates between opposing body parts. Sometimes you'll do an upper-body exercise followed by a lower; others times, you'll do a pressing movement followed by a pulling one.

By setting things up this way, you are not in danger of reaching muscular fatigue early in the workout; instead, you'll be challenged both anaerobically *and* aerobically—meaning you will work your muscles and your cardiovascular system. This leads to an increase in something called EPOC, *or* excess post-exercise oxygen consumption.

As the name implies, EPOC is a measured increase in the rate of oxygen intake following strenuous exercise. In recovery, oxygen facilitates a number of processes that adapt the body to the exercise just performed (such as cellular repair, muscle growth, and hormonal optimization), so increased oxygen consumption can speed those processes. Another use of EPOC is to fuel the increased metabolism from exercise-induced increases in body temperature.

All of that is a really long way of saying that metabolic resistance training has been shown to drastically and rapidly increase metabolism, making it exceptional for fat loss.

Metabolic resistance training has also been shown as one of the best ways to increase insulin sensitivity. While it is true that all weight training helps insulin sensitivity, two separate studies published in the *Journal of Strength and Conditioning Research* have specifically demonstrated that the effect of metabolic resistance training on insulin sensitivity is greater than with other training modalities.

Each workout in Phase I will consist of two or three metabolic resistance circuits, each of which will be made up of as many as five exercises.

Nutrition Program

Your dietary prescriptions for Prime are some of the most effective and thoroughly researched methods ever discussed. As with all other phases, Prime focuses on intermittent fasting and carb cycling, with an added twist: the insulin reset.

The insulin reset is pretty much what it sounds like: a specific dietary protocol intended to reset your insulin sensitivity. The insulin reset utilizes carb cycling in the sense that you're always eating more carbs on workout days—however, this starts out in a relatively intense fashion: with *zero* carbs three days per week.

During the first two weeks of Prime, you will take in no carbohydrates whatsoever on the days that you don't train with weights. On days you do train, you're limited to 30 grams. We recommend that all 30 grams of carbs come in the form of a post-workout shake.

Although it's not exactly fun eliminating carbs for a couple weeks, it's incredibly effective and surprisingly easy to adjust to. This is not a gimmick. While some diets will put you through a crash course of low carbs where you lose water weight and *appear* to have a lot of success only to put it right back on, this is the first phase of a complex scientific strategy designed to keep the weight off. More carbs will be added after the first two weeks, and you won't become fatter. And as you progress, you'll see that more and more carbs will continue to be added because your insulin will be better able to use those carbs to create a muscle-building and fat-burning environment.

And, if you think that this level of carb reduction sounds extreme, keep in mind that technically it's not zero carbs. You will be eating plenty of fibrous vegetables that we consider "free foods." These foods—when combined with the amount of fat and protein you'll be eating—will keep you much fuller than you'd ever imagine on a "zero-carb" plan.

We restrict carbohydrate intake to very low levels for these first two weeks because it's the fastest way to get your insulin under control. As you know, when you're minimizing carbs, you're also minimizing the secretion of insulin. Keeping insulin levels low will help your body become *more* sensitive to it—which means that you'll need less to get the job done by the second phase of the program. That would be impressive enough on its own, but what's more, this first phase is what stabilizes your blood sugar to allow for you to cheat with all your favorite foods later in the program.

While creating an environment that encourages insulin sensitivity is great, it's equally important to nurture that environment. In other words, you can't avoid carbs forever.* However, you can't just go back to pounding doughnuts and expect to keep your newfound insulin sensitivity. Not yet, at least—the rebound effect would be too great, and in addition to messing up your insulin management again, you'd also gain back any weight that you'd lost up till that point.

For this reason, the second half of Prime focuses on carb reintroduction.

During weeks three and four of Phase I, you will close out your insulin reset by slowly bringing carbs back into your diet, starting with the most important time: post-workout.

For week three, you'll still be eating zero carbs on non-workout days, but on training days, you're going to take in 75 grams of carbs, all of which will be consumed within three hours after finishing your workout. Now, 75 grams isn't much, but you'll be surprised at how different you feel taking in carbs, particularly in terms of recovery. Most of these 75 grams should come from your post-workout shake, with the remainder coming from starchy carbs like sweet potatoes.

---

* Well, you probably *could* avoid carbs forever, but life wouldn't be as much fun. That means avoiding beer, ice cream, and especially beer-flavored ice cream. Yeah. That's a thing.

During the final week of Prime, you'll be earning another notch. On non-workout days, you'll take in up to 50 grams of carbs, and on workout days, you get a whopping 100 grams. This allows you to have both a post-workout shake and a secondary source of carbs.

MEAL TIMING AND STRUCTURE

Fasting

During Prime, you'll be using what you'll call the 16/8.* We'd love to tell you that the 16/8 is a delicious sub sandwich with eight meats and sixteen toppings, but in fact it just means that you will fast for sixteen out of every twenty-four hours, with the remaining eight hours being your feeding window.

While in some sense it won't make a huge difference how you structure that breakdown, we recommend setting your feeding window to begin anywhere between noon (ending at eight P.M.) and five P.M. (ending at one A.M.), depending on when you wake up and go to bed. Put another way, you should look to have your first meal about six to eight hours after you wake up, but this isn't a hard rule.** Remember, this eating structure is flexible.

The number of meals you eat during this time period is up to you, so whether it's two or five meals doesn't matter. Your only focus is eating by the clock. Plus, you can shift your eating window. So if one day you want to start eating at noon and the next you want to eat at three P.M., it's fine—as long as you still end up fasting for sixteen hours and eating for eight.

Training and Nutrient Timing

You'll be eating your carbohydrates later in the day in order to maximize the effects of your naturally higher insulin sensitivity. On non-workout days, eat these carbs three to four hours before you go to bed. (If you go to bed at ten P.M., don't eat carbs before six P.M.) Your meals prior to this will consist of protein and fat.

On workout days, it's best to have carbs after your workout; for this reason, we recommend training a bit later in the day. Your first meal of the day should consist of protein and fat and would ideally take place about three to four hours before your workout. Your next meal would be immediately after your workout, and all the allotted carbs for the day should be eaten then.

---

* We have to tip our hats to Martin Berkhan. Not only is he the originator of the 16/8 method, but he is also largely responsible for the recent recognition of intermittent fasting as a credible dietary strategy as well as a driving force behind the entire intermittent fasting movement.

** Speaking generally, fasting is easier earlier in the day than later. We do not, for example, recommend starting your feeding window when you wake up at six A.M. and ending at two P.M. That's a recipe for disaster; psychologically, it's much easier to wait until you're allowed to eat than it is to stop eating once you've already started. But if that's your preference, it can be done.

EATING 101: FOOD CHOICES
AND HOW TO BUILD YOUR MEALS

We want to make your new style of eating as simple as possible. We know that there will be an adjustment period, but this approach should be the least restrictive diet you've ever tried. For that reason, you have all the freedom to choose the foods you want. In this section we provide an extensive list of foods to choose from to satisfy meal composition and macronutrient requirements during the various phases in this program.

As should be very clear by now, our utmost goal is to teach you as much as possible about training and nutrition over the course of the program. This way, when you are no longer our Padawan,* you will be able to maintain your new physique by instinct, knowledge, and familiarity.

To that end, while we'll give you a few examples of meals, we are literally giving you all the tools necessary to create healthy, physique-friendly meals for yourself, every single day. Remember, part of being Alpha is being self-sufficient—and the ability to feed yourself is a basic human function that has been lost on the men of the world. As an Alpha, it'll be your job to help reverse the trend. (You should probably learn how to cook, too, but that's another book altogether.)

At this time, we would like to introduce you to your new favorite thing: MyPlate by Livestrong.com (www.livestrong.com/myplate). Livestrong.com has one of the most comprehensive food databases in the world, including listings for every food we include on the following lists—and nearly every food we didn't! MyPlate uses that database to tell you the breakdown of the nutritional content.

For any food you select from the list (or elsewhere), simply go to the website and type in the name of the food and how much you ate; MyPlate will do the rest. In addition to telling you the calorie content and exactly how many grams of carbs, fat, and protein are in the food, MyPlate can act as your food journal—just set up an account (it's free), and you can save your meals.

In order to get the most accurate information, you will need to measure your food, either by weighing it on a food scale (recommended) or making a general estimate (don't be so lazy). Sure, this is a pain in the ass for the first week or so, but it's a process that has tremendous long-term benefit: by creating your meals in this way, you will begin to develop

* Padawan *is the official term for a Jedi apprentice. If you haven't figured it out by now, we are huge fucking nerds, and we love us some* Star Wars.

an uncanny sense of what a serving size should look like for your body and your goals, even as they change.

Think of yourself as Daniel-san in The Karate Kid—*we're like Mr. Miyagi, making you do seemingly mundane and pointless tasks, but just when you're thinking we've been wasting your time going all wax-on, wax-off, it turns out—bam—we taught you karate.* Yeah, that's basically what's going on here.*

We should mention that if you're consuming a food that has nutrition information on the package, there's no need to check the site—always rely on that information for the most accurate nutrition facts. But you should still go ahead and log it on the site for your records.

Finally, please *recognize that for reasons pertaining equally to sanity and spatial constraints, we can't list every food you can eat—that's what MyPlate is for. The lists below cover only a fraction of the foods you can eat while on the program; these are just a few dozen items of each type that we eat regularly. Keep in mind that the nutritional guidelines are less concerned with* what *you eat than they are with* when *you eat it.*

Engineering the Alpha was designed this way so that people of any *dietary discipline can do the program. Whether you're paleo or vegan, gluten free or a pescatarian, as long as you get the correct number of calories and each macronutrient, and you stick to the meal-timing recommendations, you can eat whatever you like. Within reason.***

We're giving you a lot of autonomy here, so be smart and make Alpha decisions.

■ CALORIE AND MACRONUTRIENT REQUIREMENTS (OR, HOW MUCH TO EAT)

Determining Your Daily Calories

First, we need to figure out your daily caloric need—the basic food intake you'd need to stay exactly as you are now. Obviously, this is just a starting point that we will manipulate to transform you into an Alpha.

There are all sorts of formulas to determine this (most are not very good), and it's important to recognize that no calorie formula is perfect. But having a formula that helps you determine how much you should be eating is one of the most effective ways to keep you on

---

* *Miyagi the mentor leading Daniel the hero through a series of tests on the Road of Trials; the resulting ability to defend himself is both the magic weapon and the ultimate boon. Campbell is everywhere. We're not making this up.*

** *A more extreme version of this dietary approach is IIFYM, or If It Fits Your Macros, popularized by Alan Aragon and Layne Norton, two nutritional wizards whom we would like to honor with a bro-fist.*

track without confusion. To that end, Roman has spent the last ten years testing and tweaking custom calorie formulas to come up with a chart that we have found to be exponentially more accurate and effective for fat loss than the others.

To determine your maintenance caloric intake for Engineering the Alpha, we'll be using the following chart:

Current Body Fat	Maintenance Caloric Intake (calories per pound of LBM)
6%–12%	17
12.1%–15%	16
15.1%–19%	15
19.1%–22%	14
22.1% or above	13

To use the above chart, you must first find out your body fat percentage and your LBM. As a reminder, here's how to figure your LBM:

1. Figure out your body fat percentage.

2. Subtract your body fat percentage from 100. This is your fat-free mass.

3. Multiply your fat-free mass (as a percentage) by your body weight. This result is your LBM.

Now, looking at the chart, you see a pretty big range; someone with low body fat is going to eat more calories than someone with very high body fat. The reason for this is rate of fat loss—the more fat you have on your body, the faster you can lose it. Moreover, the more of it you can lose without sacrificing LBM. Therefore, you can consume fewer calories and still have a great rate of fat loss without really affecting the metabolic processes responsible for losing fat and gaining lean muscle. After all, if you go too low on calories, your fat loss can slow to a crawl and gaining muscle can become increasingly difficult. It's the whole reason why we're making sure your hormones are optimized so your body can make the types of changes that you want to experience.

In any event, once you know your body fat and LBM, simply find your percentage on the chart and multiply the corresponding number by your LBM. This number is your mainte- nance caloric intake.

Let's take your average two-hundred-pound guy who is 20 percent body fat. We'll call this man Steve.

200 pounds x 20% body fat = 40 pounds of body fat

200 pounds – 40 pounds of fat = 160 pounds of LBM

160 x 14 (because our 200-pounder is between 19 and 22 percent body fat) = 2,240 calories per day for Steve

■ PRIME: THE DIET

Determine Your Daily Caloric Intake During Prime

Of course, you're not interested in maintaining; you want to lose fat and gain muscle—during Prime, you're going to achieve the former and set yourself up for the latter.

For this phase, you're going to adjust your daily caloric intake as follows:

- *To determine your calories for workout days, subtract 300 from your maintenance calories.*
- *To determine your calories for non-workout days, subtract 500 calories.*

So Steve would be eating 1,940 calories per day on workout days and 1,740 on non-workout days.

Once you've done that, we can move on to figuring out how much of each macronutrient to eat.

■ MACRONUTRIENT BREAKDOWN

Protein

Protein intake is determined by your lean body mass, and during this phase you'll be eating less protein than at any other time of the program. One of the goals of Prime is to minimize insulin production, and eating too much protein can actually create an insulin spike. That's because the amino acids in protein can signal your pancreas to produce insulin.[*]

Protein intake will be set as follows:

Workout days: 0.8 grams protein per pound of LBM

Non-workout days: 0.7 grams protein per pound of LBM

Let's use Steve as an example again. Remember, our two-hundred-pound man with 20 percent body fat has an LBM of 160 pounds. Given that information:

160 x 0.8 = 128 grams of protein on workout days

160 x 0.7 = 112 grams of protein on non-workout days

---

[*] *The term for this is* gluconeogenesis. *We haven't had any science terms in a while, so this seemed like a good time to throw that in.*

Protein has 4 calories per gram, so that works out to 512 calories from protein on work-out days. If you want to think of calories like a bank account, here's where Steve would currently stand on workout days:

Beginning balance: 1,940 calories

Protein: –512 calories

Remaining balance: 1,428 calories

Carbs

We've already discussed carbs in a general sense, but let's look at them in terms of calories. Like protein, carbohydrates have 4 calories per gram.

So during Prime that would look like this:

Weeks 1–2

- Workout days: 30 grams (120 calories)
- Non-workout days: 0 grams (0 calories)

Week 3

- Workout days: 75 grams (300 calories)
- Non-workout days: 0 grams (0 calories)

Week 4

- Workout days: 100 grams (400 calories)
- Non-workout days: 50 grams (200 calories)

Going back to Steve's calorie balance on training days:

Beginning balance: 1,940 calories

Protein: –512 calories

Carbs: –120 calories

Remaining balance: 1,308 calories

Fat

At this point, you know your daily calories and have subtracted the caloric values of both your protein consumption and your carb intake. Now, you still have a balance of a few hun-dred calories; these will come from fat sources—and yes, that generally equates to a lot of fat. But, as you know by now, if you're getting healthy fats from quality sources like steak, eggs, and salmon, you're taking another step on the path toward hormonal optimization.

Fat has 9 calories per gram, so take your remaining balance of calories and divide by 9. The result is how many grams of fat you eat. Let's look at Steve's workout day example again. After subtracting calories from protein and carbs, he's got 1,308 calories left:

1,308 calories / 9 = 145 grams of fat

■ THE ALPHA EATING GUIDE

You want to know what to eat? Good, because we want to feed you—and make sure this plan has you feeling free, flexible, and ready to feast. Here is our Alpha-approved shopping list. Stock up on these foods, and then plug and play each option into the meal guides. The foods have been split into categories: proteins, free veggies, fats, and carbs. While we'll provide you with very specific numbers, we'll also show you how to create your own meal plan so every day can offer a menu loaded with your favorites. Dig in.

PROTEINS					
Beef	**Poultry**	**Pork and Lamb**	**Shellfish**	**Fishies**	**Eggies and Dairy**
Brisket	Chicken, Breast	Canadian Bacon	Clams	Anchovy	Egg White
Chuck, Arm Pot Roast	Chicken, Leg	Ham, Fresh, 95% Lean	Crab	Bluefish	Cottage Cheese, Nonfat
Cured, Dried Beef	Chicken, Thigh	Lamb, Leg, Chop	Lobster	Cod	Mozzarella Cheese, Nonfat
Eye Round	Chicken, Wing	Pork Chop, Sirloin, Boneless	Oysters	Flounder, Sole	Protein Powder (Biotrust Protein)
Filet Mignon	Turkey, Breast	Pork Loin	Scallops	Haddock	Whole Egg
Flank Steak	Turkey, Leg	Pork Tenderloin	Shrimp	Halibut	
Ground Beef, 95% Lean	Turkey Sausage			Herring	
New York Strip				Mackerel	
Rib Eye				Orange Roughy	
Sirloin				Salmon	
Skirt Steak				Sea Bass	
				Snapper	
				Swordfish	
				Tilapia	
				Tuna, Canned	
				Tuna, Fresh	

FREE VEGETABLES						
These veggies can be eaten anytime and added to any meal. Veggies should be added to at least three meals daily.						
Arugula	Asparagus	Broccoli	Brussels Sprouts	Cabbage	Cauliflower	Cucumber
Eggplant	Lettuce	Mushroom	Okra	Onion	Peppers	Radish
Snow Peas	Spinach	Tomato	Watercress	Zucchini		

FATS

Eggies and Dairy	Oils*	Nuts and Seeds*	Fruits and Veggies
Block Cheese (American, Cheddar, Colby, etc.)	Canola Oil	Almonds, Almond Butter	Avocado
Butter	Coconut Oil	Brazil Nuts	Olives
Cream Cheese	Extra-Virgin Olive Oil	Cashews, Cashew Butter	
Feta Cheese	Fish Oil Capsules	Flaxseeds (must consume ground, not whole)	
Mozzarella Cheese, Whole Milk	Flaxseed Oil	Hazelnuts	
Parmesan Cheese, Grated	Hemp Oil	Pecans	
Ricotta Cheese, Whole Milk	Krill Oil (Prograde EFA Icon)	Pistachios	
Sour Cream	Primrose Oil	Pumpkin Seeds	
Whole Egg	Pumpkin Seed Oil	Sunflower Seeds	
	All oils are 14g fat, 0g protein, 0g carb.	Walnuts	
		All nuts and seeds should be either dry roasted or raw (not cooked in oil). Raw nuts can be purchased at your local health food store.	

LOW-GI/GL CARBS (These carbs are allowed in any P+C meal.)

Legumes	Fruits	Veggies	Whole-Grain Breads*	Other Grains
Black Beans	Apple	Artichoke	100% Whole-Wheat	Barley
Black-Eyed Peas	Apricot	Beets	Multigrain	Buckwheat
Chickpeas	Blackberries	Carrots	Oat Bran	Cream of Rice
Green Peas	Blueberries	Pumpkin	Pita, 100% Whole-Wheat	Oat Bran
Kidney Beans	Cantaloupe	Rutabaga	Pumpernickel	Oatmeal
Lentils	Cherries	Squash	Rye	Quinoa
Lima Beans	Cranberries	Sweet Potato	Tortilla Wrap, 100% Whole-Wheat	Rice: Brown, Jasmine, or White
Navy Beans	Grapefruit	Yam	Tortilla Wrap, 100% Whole-Wheat, Low-Carb, High-Fiber	
Pinto Beans	Grapes			
White Beans	Honeydew		*See package to ensure the most accurate nutrition information.*	
	Kiwi			
	Mango			
	Orange			
	Peach			
	Pear			
	Pineapple			
	Plum			
	Raspberries			
	Rhubarb			
	Strawberries			
	Watermelon			

■ THE ALPHA EATING EQUATION: PRIME

Workout Days

—Using the information in the chart, figure out how many calories you need in order to maintain your body weight.

—Subtract 300 from that number. Now we've got your calories for workout days.

—Multiply your lean body mass by 0.8. This number represents how much protein you should eat.

—Based on where you are in Prime, set carbs at either 30, 75, or 100.

—Take your total grams of protein and your total grams of carbs, and add them together.

—Multiply that number by 4. This gives you the total number of calories from protein and carbs.

—Subtract this number from your calories for workout days. This number is how many calories from fat you need.

—Divide this number by 9. This is how many grams of fat you need.

Because numbers can be tricky, let's make sure we're not letting math stand in the way. Let's use Steve as an example. If you remember, Steve is two hundred pounds with 20 percent body fat and an LBM of 160 pounds.

Daily calories = 2,240
2,240 – 300 = 1,940 calories on training days
160 x 0.8 = 128 grams of protein
Carbs = 30 grams (Prime, week 1)
128 (grams of protein) + 30 (grams of carbs) = 158
158 x 4 = 632 calories
1,940 – 632 = 1,308 calories from fat
1,308 / 9 = 145 grams of fat per day

Total goal numbers for week 1 Prime, workout days:

1,940 calories | 128 grams of protein | 30 grams of carbs | 145 grams of fat

Non-Workout Days

We repeat the same process for non-workout days:

—Using the information in the chart, figure out how many calories you need in order to maintain your body weight.

—Subtract 500 from that number. Now we've got your calories for non-workout days.

—Multiply your lean body mass by 0.7. This number represents how much protein you should eat.

—Based on where you are in Prime, set carbs at either 0 or 50.

—Take your total grams of protein and your total grams of carbs, and add them together.

—Multiply that number by 4. This gives you the total number of calories from protein and carbs.

—Subtract this number from your calories for non-workout days. This number is how many calories from fat you need.

—Divide this number by 9. This is how many grams of fat you need.

Example using a two-hundred-pound man with 20 percent body fat and an LBM of 160 pounds:

Daily calories = 2,240
2,240 – 500 = 1,740 calories on non-workout days
160 x 0.7 = 112 grams of protein
Carbs = 0 grams (Prime, week 1)
112 (grams of protein) + 0 (grams of carbs) = 112
112 x 4 = 448 calories
1,740 – 448 = 1,292 calories from fat
1,292 / 9 = 143 grams of fat per day

Total goal numbers for week 1 Prime, non-workout days:

1,740 calories │ 112 grams of protein │ 0 grams of carbs │ 143 grams of fat

That's that.

Now you have a comprehensive guide for your nutrition—just follow the steps and you'll quickly see how simple it is. After all, it's just a little math. And who doesn't love math, right? Right?

With all that covered, let's move on to the workouts for Phase I.

SAMPLE MEAL PLAN (ROMAN'S NUTRITION GUIDE)

To make things as relatable as possible, it's probably helpful if we give you a real world example. This is the exact plan Roman used during the process of writing this book.

Weighing 192 pounds with 8 percent body fat, Roman has 15.36 pounds of fat on his body, leaving him with 176.64 pounds of lean body mass. Using the chart, we multiplied his LBM by 17 to get his maintenance calories of 3,003.

Based on that information, the following two pages show a sample of his diet, as well as a sample of what Steve's diet could look like during Prime.

ROMAN: **Phase I Meal Plan for Workout Days**

Contents	Protein (grams)	Carbs (grams)	Fats (grams)	Calories
First Solid Meal P+F 8 eggs, 1 medium avocado, 2 tbsp coconut oil, cooked spinach or kale	48	0	96	1056
Para-Workout Beverage P+C Workout Beverage—3 scoops BioTrust Low-Carb mixed with 12 oz fat-free milk. Consume ⅔ of this drink during the second half of your workout. Finish immediately upon completion.	50	30	5	365
Dinner Meal P+C+F 5 oz rib eye cooked in 3.5 tbsp organic butter, 1 cup sweet potato, ½ cup mixed nuts	44	70	96	1320
Daily Totals	**142**	**100**	**197**	**2741**

ROMAN: **Phase I Meal Plan for Non-Workout Days**

Contents	Protein (grams)	Carbs (grams)	Fats (grams)	Calories
First Solid Meal P+F 3 slices Canadian bacon, extra lean (90%) ground beef, 2 tbsp coconut oil (cooking), 2 tbsp heavy cream in coffee or tea	42	0	60	708
Midday Meal P+C+F Lean meat (turkey, chicken, fillet), 1 cup mixed berries, 1 oz almonds, mixed greens salad, 3 tbsp extra-virgin olive oil and balsamic vinegar	42	20	65	833
Dinner Meal P+C+F Cooked salmon fillet, 2 boiled red potatoes with organic butter, 2 squares dark chocolate, steamed and seasoned broccoli	42	30	80	1008
Daily Totals	**126**	**50**	**205**	**2549**

STEVE: Phase I Meal Plan for Workout Days

Contents	Protein (grams)	Carbs (grams)	Fats (grams)	Calories
First Solid Meal P+F 6 eggs, ½ medium avocado, 2 tablespoons coconut oil, cooked spinach or kale	39	0	54	642
Para-Workout Beverage P+C Workout Beverage—3 scoops BioTrust Low-Carb mixed with 12 oz fat-free milk. Consume ⅔ of this drink during the second half of your workout. Finish immediately upon completion.	50	30	5	365
Dinner Meal P+C+F 5 oz rib eye cooked in organic butter, 1 cup sweet potato, ¼ cup mixed nuts	39	70	55	931
Daily Totals	**128**	**100**	**145**	**1938**

STEVE: Phase I Meal Plan for Non-Workout Days

Contents	Protein (grams)	Carbs (grams)	Fats (grams)	Calories
First Solid Meal P+F 2 slices Canadian bacon, extra lean (90%) ground beef, 1 tbsp coconut oil (cooking), 1 tbsp heavy cream in coffee or tea	37	0	40	508
Midday Meal P+C+F Lean meat (turkey, chicken, fillet), 1 cup mixed berries, 1 oz almonds, mixed greens salad, 1 tbsp extra-virgin olive oil and balsamic vinegar	37	20	40	588
Dinner Meal P+C+F Cooked salmon fillet, 2 boiled red potatoes with organic butter, 1 square dark chocolate, steamed and seasoned broccoli	38	30	41	641
Daily Totals	**112**	**50**	**143**	**1737**

PHASE I WORKOUTS

If your diet is the engine that drives hormonal optimization, then the workouts are the high-performance fuel that makes everything work much more efficiently. Your first phase of training consists of four different workouts. Each workout is a full-body routine that primarily focuses on compound exercises to work multiple muscles at the same time. These exercises will be the foundation of all the workouts you perform on this entire program, but the variations will become more difficult as you progress. The workouts have been set up in a way that keeps your body guessing which routine comes next. At the same time, each workout is similar and based on time, which allows you to see progression throughout the phase. After all, that's the primary goal of any workout: to show improvement every session. Try to increase your weight each week, and you'll be well on your way to a new body by the time Phase II begins.

Use the schedule below to determine when you'll perform each of the workouts. We've provided you with a simple template that starts on Monday. If you choose to start on a different day, just make sure you follow the same pattern of workout days and rest days. That is, if you start Workout 1 on Tuesday, just push the schedule back one day.

Prime Training Schedule							
	Monday	Tuesday	Wednesday	Thursday	Friday	Saturday	Sunday
Week 1	Workout 1	Workout 2	OFF	Workout 3	Workout 4	OFF	OFF
Week 2	Workout 3	Workout 1	OFF	Workout 4	Workout 2	OFF	OFF
Week 3	Workout 4	Workout 3	OFF	Workout 2	Workout 1	OFF	OFF
Week 4	Workout 2	Workout 4	OFF	Workout 1	Workout 3	OFF	OFF

HOW TO SPOT AN ALPHA IN THE GYM: PART I

Through the four phases, you'll notice a few unique exercises. We consider these a special part of Engineering the Alpha. Not only will these movements help you build a better body, but they will allow you to distinguish other Alphas in the gym. In Prime, we introduce you to the first Alpha exercise: the Javelin Press.

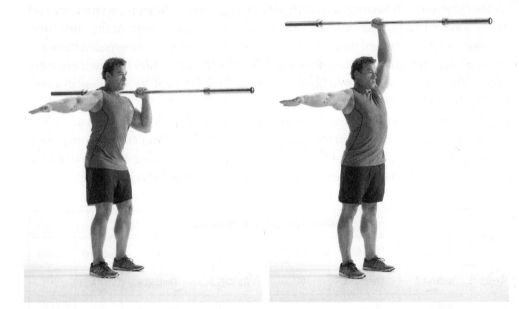

◗ Hold a barbell at shoulder level with your hand in the middle of the barbell. Hold the other arm straight out to the side.

◗ Brace your abs and press your arm straight up, making sure to stabilize at the trunk and the shoulder.

◗ Your body should not tilt one way or the other, and the barbell should remain level.

◗ Softly lock your arm at the top of the movement.

◗ Slowly return to the starting position.

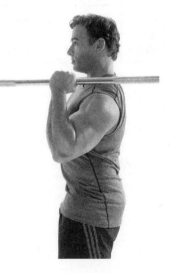

PHASE I, WORKOUT 1

A1 **Goblet Squat**
10–12 reps

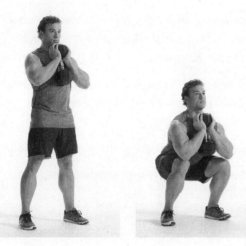

◗ Hold a dumbbell vertically next to your chest, with both hands cupping the dumbbell head.

◗ Push your hips back and lower your body into a squat until your upper thighs are at least parallel to the floor. Your elbows should brush the insides of your knees in the bottom position.

◗ Pause, then press your body back up.

A2 **Incline Dumbbell Chest Press**
8–10 reps

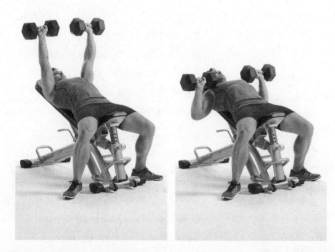

◗ Set an adjustable bench to an incline of 30 to 45 degrees.

◗ Grab a pair of dumbbells and lie faceup on the bench. Hold the dumbbells directly above your shoulders with your arms straight.

◗ Lower the dumbbells to the sides of your chest, pause, and then press the weights back above your chest.

A3 **Single-Arm Dumbbell Row**
8 reps per arm

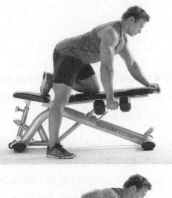

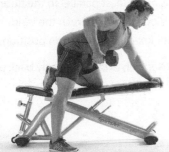

♦ Grab a dumbbell in your right hand.

♦ Push your hips back and bend over until your torso is almost parallel to the floor. Place your left hand on a bench in front of your body. Your right arm should hang at arm's length with your palm facing your other arm.

♦ Keeping your elbow close to your body, pull the dumbbell up to your chest by squeezing your shoulder blade back.

♦ Pause, then lower back to the starting position.

♦ Complete all prescribed reps, then switch arms and repeat.

A4 **Kettlebell Romanian Deadlift**
12–15 reps

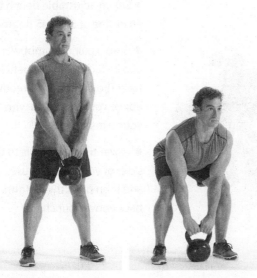

♦ Grab a kettlebell, and hold it at arm's length in front of your thighs. Stand with your feet hip-width apart and your knees slightly bent.

♦ Without changing the bend in your knees, bend at your hips and lower your torso until it's almost parallel to the floor.

♦ Pause, then raise your torso back to the starting position.

A5 Plank
30 seconds

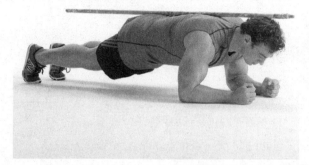

◗ Start to get in a push-up position, but bend your elbows and rest your weight on your forearms instead of on your hands. Your body should form a straight line from your shoulders to your ankles.

◗ Brace your core by contracting your abs as if you were about to be punched in the gut.

◗ Hold this position as directed.

Perform A1–A5 in a circuit fashion, resting no more than 30 seconds between exercises. Perform 4 circuits, resting 3 minutes between each. After your last set, rest 2 minutes and proceed to the next circuit.

B1 Chin-Up
As many as possible

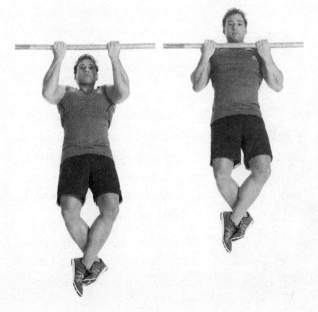

◗ Grab a chin-up bar with a shoulder-width underhand grip.

◗ Hang at arm's length and pull your shoulder blades down and back so that your shoulders are as far from your ears as possible.

◗ Pull your chest to the bar as you squeeze your shoulder blades together.

◗ Pause, and then lower your body back to the starting position.

B2 Body-Weight Glute Bridge
12 reps

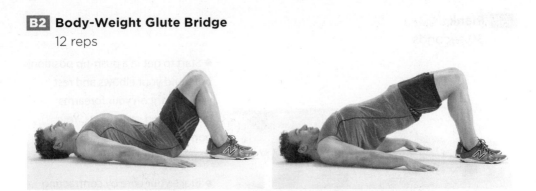

◆ Lie faceup on the floor with your knees bent and your feet flat on the floor.

◆ Raise your hips so your body forms a straight line from your shoulders to your knees.

◆ Pause in the up position, then lower your body back to the starting position.

B3 Body-Weight Reverse Lunge
8 reps per leg

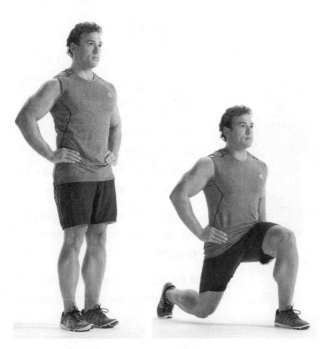

◆ Place your hands on your hips, pull your shoulders back, and stand as tall as you can.

◆ Step backward with your right leg and slowly lower your body until your front knee is bent at least 90 degrees.

◆ Pause, then push yourself to the starting position as quickly as you can.

◆ Complete the prescribed number of reps with your right leg, then do the same number with your left leg.

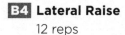 **Lateral Raise**
12 reps

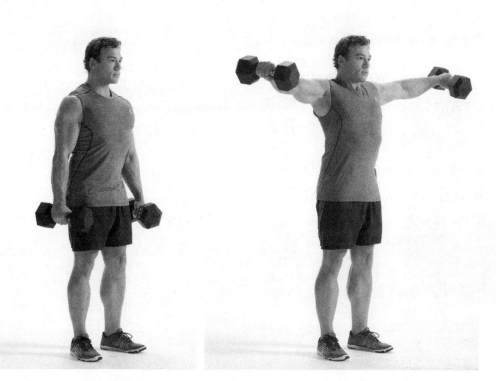

◗ Grab a pair of dumbbells and stand tall with a slight bend in your knees. Your arms should hang straight down from your shoulders with your elbows slightly bent.

◗ Hold your body still and raise your arms out to the sides until your hands are in line with your shoulders.

◗ Pause, then return to the starting position.

Perform B1–B4 in a circuit fashion, resting no more than 20 seconds between exercises. Perform 3 circuits, resting 90 seconds between each.

PHASE I, WORKOUT 2

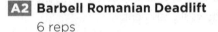 **Dumbbell Overhead Press**
8 reps

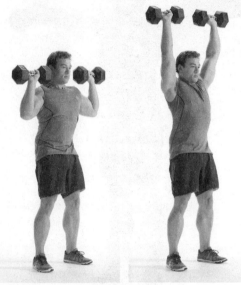

◗ Grab a pair of dumbbells and hold them just outside your shoulders with your palms facing forward.

◗ Press the weight overhead until your arms are completely straight.

◗ Pause, then slowly lower the dumbbells back to the starting position.

A2 **Barbell Romanian Deadlift**
6 reps

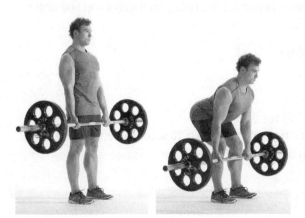

◗ Grab a barbell with an overhand grip that's just beyond shoulder-width and hold it at arm's length in front of your hips. Your knees should be slightly bent and chest pushed out. This is the starting position.

◗ Without changing the bend in your knees, bend at your hips and lower your torso until it's almost parallel to the floor.

◗ Pause, then raise your torso back to the starting position.

A3 Barbell Bent-Over Row
8 reps

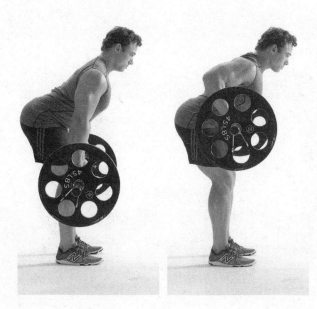

◗ Grab a barbell with an overhand grip with your hands about shoulder-width apart.

◗ Hold the bar at arm's length, and then bend at your hips and lower your torso until it's almost parallel to the floor. Your knees should be slightly bent and your lower back naturally arched.

◗ Squeeze your shoulder blades together and pull the bar up to your upper abs.

◗ Pause, then return the bar back to the starting position.

A4 Hanging Knee Raise
10 reps

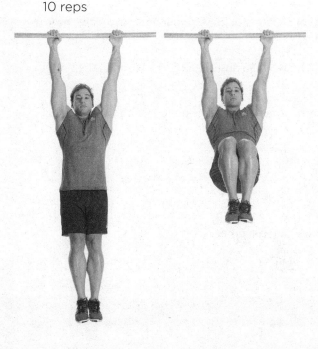

◗ Grab a chin-up bar with an overhand, shoulder-width grip. If this is too hard, set up elbow straps and hang from the bar.

◗ With your feet together and knees slightly bent, raise your hips and lift your thighs toward your chest.

◗ Stop when the top of your thighs are just above parallel to the floor, pause, and then lower your legs back to the starting position.

A5 Body-Weight Bulgarian Split Squat
8 reps per leg

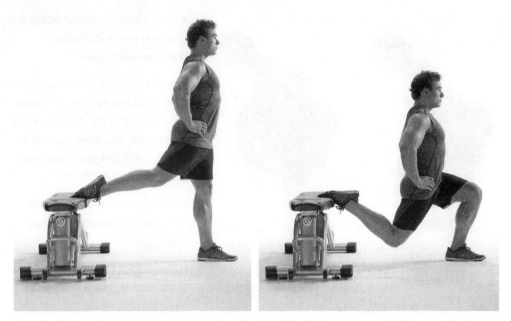

◗ Stand tall and place your hands on your hips and pull your elbows back so that your chest is up.

◗ Stand in a staggered stance with your left foot in front of your right, and place the instep of your back foot on a bench.

◗ Lower your body as far as you can, pause, then push your body back up to the starting position.

◗ Do all reps with your left foot forward, then do the same number with your right foot in front of your left.

Perform A1–A5 in a circuit fashion, resting no more than 30 seconds between exercises. Perform 5 circuits, resting 3 minutes between each.

B Two-Arm Kettlebell Swing
30–45 seconds

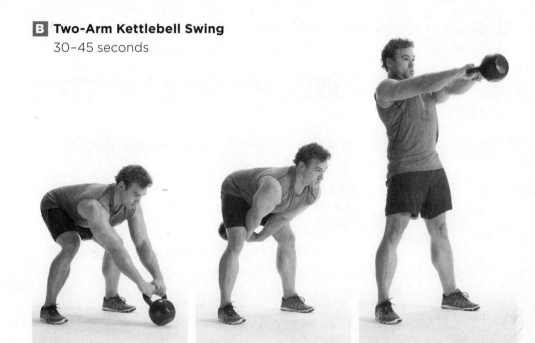

● Grab a kettlebell with both hands with an overhand grip and hold it in front of your waist at arm's length. Set your feet slightly wider than shoulder-width apart.

● Keeping your lower back slightly arched, bend at your hips and knees, and lower your torso until it forms a 45-degree angle to the floor.

● Now swing the kettlebell between your legs. Keeping your arms straight, thrust your hips forward, straighten your knees, and swing the kettlebell up to chest level as you rise to standing position.

● Reverse the movement and swing the kettlebell back between your legs again.
That's 1 rep.

Perform 3 sets of Kettlebell Swings, resting 2 minutes between each. After your last set, rest 2 minutes and proceed to the next circuit.

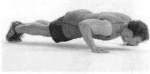

C1 Push-Up
12–15 reps

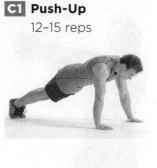

◗ Get on all fours, and place your hands on the floor slightly wider than and in line with your shoulders. Your body should form a straight line from your ankles to your shoulders.

◗ Squeeze your abs as tight as possible and keep them contracted for the entire exercise.

◗ Lower your body until your chest nearly touches the floor, making sure that you tuck your elbows close to the sides of your torso.

◗ Pause, then push yourself back to the starting position.

C2 Jump Squat
10 reps

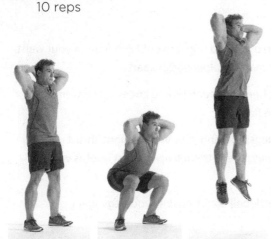

◗ Place your fingers on the back of your head and pull your elbows back so that they're in line with your body.

◗ Dip your knees in preparation to leap.

◗ Explosively jump as high as you can, while keeping your hands behind your head as you jump.

◗ When you land, immediately squat down and jump again.

C3 Plank
30 seconds

Perform C1–C3 in a circuit fashion, resting no more than 15 seconds between exercises. Perform 2 circuits, resting 30 seconds between circuits.

PHASE I, WORKOUT 3

A Barbell Deadlift
6–8 reps

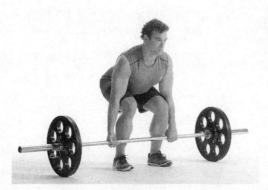

◗ Load a barbell and roll it up against your shins.

◗ Bend at your hips and knees, and grab the bar with an overhand grip that's about shoulder-width.

◗ Without allowing your lower back to round, stand up, thrust your hips forward, and squeeze your glutes.

◗ Pause, then lower the bar back to the floor while keeping it as close to your body as possible.

Perform 3 sets of deadlifts, resting 3 minutes between each. Warm up slowly and work up to your actual training weight. After your last set, rest 2 minutes and proceed to the next circuit.

B1 Javelin Press
6–8 reps

B2 Goblet Squat
10 reps

B3 Inverted Row
6–10 reps

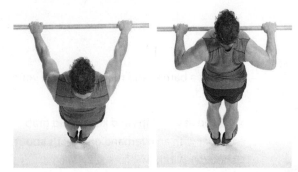

● Grab a stationary bar with an overhand, shoulder-width grip. Your arms should be straight and your body should form a straight line from your shoulders to your ankles.

● Pull your shoulder blades back and lift your body until your chest touches the bar.

● Pause, then slowly lower your body back to the starting position.

B4 Single-Leg Hip Raise
10 reps per leg

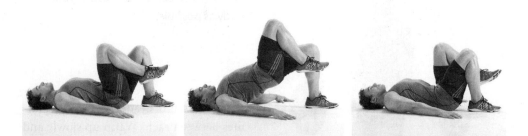

● Lie faceup on the floor with your left knee bent and your right leg straight.

● Raise your right leg until it's in line with your left thigh, and place your arms out to the sides.

● Push your hips upward, keeping your right leg elevated.

● Pause, then slowly lower your body and leg back to the starting position.

● Complete the prescribed number of reps with your right leg, then switch legs and do the same number with your left leg.

Perform B1–B4 in a circuit fashion, resting no more than 30 seconds between exercises. Perform 4 circuits, resting 90 seconds between each. After your last set, rest 2 minutes and proceed to the next circuit.

C1 Plank
Hold as long as possible

C2 Jumping Jack
As many as possible in 45 seconds

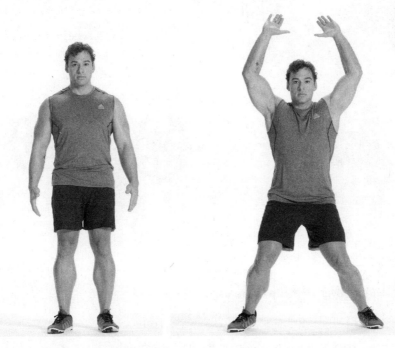

● Begin facing forward with your arms at your sides.

● Jump up slightly and spread your legs as you bring your arms together overhead.

● Jump up slightly again and return to the starting position, bringing your legs together and arms back down to your sides.

C3 Chin-Up
As many as possible

Perform C1–C3 in a circuit fashion, resting no more than 15 seconds between exercises. Perform only 1 circuit.

PHASE I, WORKOUT 4

A1 **Barbell Front Squat**
8 reps

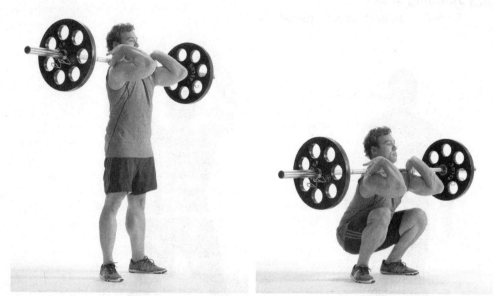

- Hold a barbell with an overhand grip that's just beyond shoulder width.

- Raise your upper arms until they're parallel to the floor.

- Allow the bar to roll back so that it's resting on the front of your shoulders.

- Lower your body until the tops of your thighs are at least parallel to the floor.

- Pause, then push your body back to the starting position.

A2 **Plank**
30 seconds

A3 **Javelin Press**
10 reps

Plank
30 seconds

Perform A1–A4 in a circuit fashion, resting no more than 30 seconds between exercises. Perform 4 circuits, resting 90 seconds between each. After your last set, rest 2 minutes and proceed to the next circuit.

B1 **Barbell Glute Bridge**
6 to 8 reps

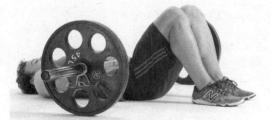

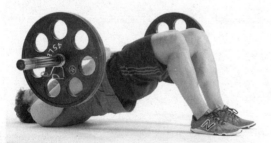

● Lay on the floor with your knees bent and feet flat on the floor.

● Put a padded barbell across your hips and grab the barbell with an overhand grip, about shoulder-width apart.

● Keeping the barbell just below your pelvis, raise your hips—while squeezing your glutes—until your hips are in line with your body.

● Return to the starting position, and repeat.

B2 **Push-Up**
As many as possible

B3 Mountain Climber
30 seconds

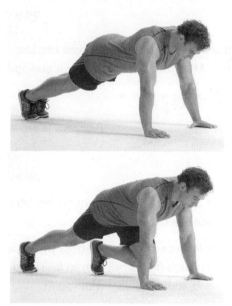

◗ Assume a push-up position with your arms completely straight. Your body should form a straight line from your shoulders to your ankles.

◗ Lift your left foot off the floor and slowly raise your knee as close to your chest as you can.

◗ Return to the starting position and repeat with your right leg.

◗ Continue alternating for the prescribed number of reps or time.

Perform B1–B3 in a circuit fashion, resting no more than 30 seconds between exercises. Perform 4 circuits, resting 90 seconds between each. After your last set, rest 2 minutes and proceed to the next circuit.

C Pull-Up
20 reps

Perform 20 total reps on the pull-up. It doesn't matter how many sets it takes as long as you get all 20. For some people, this will be 3 sets, for others, 6. Just do as many pull-ups as you can, then rest, then do more. Continue in this fashion until you get to 20. If you can get more than 10 on your first set, add some weight using a belt.

CHAPTER 10

Phase II: Adapt

EMBRACING METAMORPHOSIS

"The snake which cannot cast its skin has to die. As well, the minds which are prevented from changing their opinions, they cease to be minds."

—FRIEDRICH NIETZSCHE

Phase II of Engineering the Alpha is where things start to get really interesting, in terms of both diet and training. We'll cover diet first because, as we mentioned, you get to partake in cheat days, otherwise known as the most awesome thing to hit food since . . . well, food. It's time to master the cheat day.

But before we get to that, we want to talk about the hormonal components of Phase II. This phase is called Adapt for a few reasons: You have readapted to carbs in your diet. Your insulin receptors have adapted to a higher level of sensitivity. And, of course, your body has adapted to the workouts and dieting, making you more proficient overall.

Adapt will also be highly concerned with testosterone, a hormone so awesome that Roman got its chemical structure tattooed on his forearm.

As we explained in the hormonal breakdown discussion, testosterone is involved in everything from fat loss and muscle building to sex and confidence. During Phase II, you will notice the first results of increased testosterone.

"Oh, that's good. Write that down."

—VAN WILDER

This will happen by way of your newfound friendship with insulin. When you're insulin resistant, you store more fat, which increases estrogen and lowers testosterone; when you're insulin sensitive, you flip the switch so you lose fat, increase testosterone, and lower estrogen. Win-win.

Additionally, testosterone production will be enhanced by your training efforts. All weight training increases testosterone, but studies have shown that when you train with increased density, the effect is exacerbated. During Adapt, the training will be entirely dedicated to increasing density—and thereby testosterone.

Finally, we'll look at the hormones primarily responsible for your metabolism: leptin, T3, and T4. In order to create the context necessary to fully explain these things, let's take a look at what happens to you while you're on a diet—even an intelligent one, like the one you followed in Prime.

Overall, Adapt is about increasing your training intensity and volume so you'll not only be working harder on each set, you'll also be doing more total reps and sets. On the diet side, compared to last phase, you'll be eating *more* on training days and *less* on non-training days. And then, of course, there's cheat day, when you'll eat all types of foods that you never thought would be suggested as part of a fat-loss plan. But we not only suggest—we require you to indulge.

WHAT HAPPENS WHEN YOU DIET

The human body is amazingly proficient at adapting to the various stressors in life, including severe caloric restriction. The body quickly recognizes the caloric deficit and then promptly makes the necessary adjustments to maintain homeostasis.

This is an evolutionary adaptation that has helped our species survive in times of famine—awesome for that, but not so desirable for people who want to get lean. If you cut calories, your body will eventually adjust and hold on to more fat, which is exactly what you're trying to avoid.

We just told you that you'll be training harder, eating more on those training days, and eating less on your off days. As with everything in this book, there's a reason for our madness. When you follow a traditional diet of just eating less, this is what typically happens inside your body.

Decreased Levels of T3 and T4

T3 and T4 levels (thyroid hormones that play a major role in the regulation of metabolism) in underfed individuals mimic and can actually cause sick euthyroid syndrome. In short, low levels of these hormones are anything but desirable for individuals seeking to lose fat mass.

Decreased Basal Metabolic Rate

The overall decrease in metabolism, or basal metabolic rate, is largely due to the afore-mentioned decrease in output of T3 and T4; however, a host of other factors also contribute to the downregulation of the basal metabolic rate. In essence, metabolic rate is decelerated in an attempt to balance energy expenditure with caloric consumption, thus preserving more fat mass. So if you eat fewer calories, your body does what it can to burn fewer calories.

This effect, combined with the one above, is the reason for what we colloquially term *starvation mode*—your body thinks you're starving, and it does its best to keep you alive.

Increased Levels and Half-Life of Cortisol

Severe dieting both spikes and *extends* the half-life of cortisol. We mentioned that cortisol is a catabolic agent—when elevated for long periods of time, the catabolic effect will be directed toward your muscle. This is clearly not optimal for individuals who wish to retain lean muscle mass while attempting to lose fat. Interestingly, the serum cortisol levels associated with malnourished (underfed) individuals parallel those linked to individuals suffering from clinical depression.

Decreased Serum Leptin Levels

Generally speaking, there's a positive relationship between leptin and the amount of fat mass you're carrying. However, certain studies have shown dramatic decreases in leptin when caloric intake is highly restricted, independent of fat mass. When low levels of leptin are transmitted to the associated receptors of the hypothalamus, the hypothalamus then begins to send out various regulatory signals to the rest of the body in an attempt to decelerate fat loss and decrease energy expenditure. Or in English: low levels of leptin slow your ability to lose weight by turning your metabolism down a few notches.

It almost seems backward: the better shape you're in, the harder it is to look even better. In other words, the more you move away from the weight that your body is used to (called your set point), the more your body adapts to resist your transformation. Even though individual set points can vary greatly, one thing remains constant: the leaner you get, the worse the aforementioned problems become. But if you can change your set point by staying at a lower body fat for a longer period of time, your body will adapt and make fat loss easier—at least compared to when your body constantly lives in an overweight state.

The main reason lean people have extreme difficulty shedding that last bit of stubborn fat is that their metabolisms have hit rock bottom. Cortisol is freely running its course while T3, T4, and leptin are all slowed to a trickle, like blood to the nether regions of an eighty-year-old man in the days before Viagra.

However, there is hope—and that hope lies in cheat days.

THREE HORMONAL BENEFITS OF CHEAT DAYS

"All you need is love. But a little chocolate now and then doesn't hurt."
—CHARLES SCHULTZ

1. Increase in thyroid hormone output
When your body is in a caloric deficit, you produce less T3 and T4—both important thyroid hormones that play roles in the regulation of metabolic rate. A cheat day or strategic overfeed can help increase these hormones.

2. Increase in twenty-four-hour energy expenditure
A caloric surplus from a cheat day causes your body to increase your basal metabolic rate, which is the amount of calories you burn throughout the day. Studies have shown an increase of nearly 10 percent, and it's hypothesized that an even more significant increase is possible.

3. Increase in serum leptin levels
This might be the most important perk of cheat days from a fat-loss standpoint. Leptin levels drop when you're in a caloric deficit (lasting as little as seventy-two hours), and a periodic bump in leptin coming from a cheat day has several benefits, including increased thyroid output, increased energy expenditure and basal metabolic rate, and overall increased thermogenesis (aka fat burning).

The benefits of the cheat day are twofold. On one hand, you have the physical and physiological benefits (see "Three Hormonal Benefits of Cheat Days"). But cheat days also provide a mental and emotional break from dieting so you don't feel like you're on a diet. Most people quit diets out of frustration that they can't eat what they want. And while we're confident that the intermittent fasting structure gives you much more freedom to eat great foods, the cheat day ensures that no stone is unturned. There is a certain psychological benefit when you are able to take days off from your diet, eat whatever you want, and be confident in the knowledge that it will not make you fat.

And during the Adapt phase, you get a cheat day every single week. While there are a lot of diets that rely on cheat days to be successful, nearly any nutritional plan can, under the right set of circumstances, benefit from cheat days. So without bogging you down too much, here's a primer—the cheater's cheat sheet, if you will:

1. **Do not gorge; stop eating before you feel stuffed.** You are allowed to eat what you want but not to gorge yourself until you feel like you want to throw up.

2. **Only buy your cheat foods on your cheat day.** Then after the day is done, *get rid* of them. Remember: if it's there, you'll eat it. So throw your cheat day foods in the trash once the cheat day is over.

3. **Eat your meals and make them as cheat-y as possible.** Leave no stone unturned. Eat what you want. You certainly don't have to eat junk food; if you adhere to a gluten-free diet, you don't need to eat cookies—or you can obviously just eat gluten-free cookies. The most important things for cheat days are carbs and overall calories, so as long as you're consuming plenty of those, you can have foods that fall in line with your regular nutritional practices. *Just eat more of them.*

4. **Have fun with it.** Eat what you want without any thought of guilt. It's strategic, and it needs to be done so you can prime your body to burn more fat.

FEAST/FAST MODEL

The feast/fast model was originated by Roman in 2004, and he's been using it with his clients and his own diet ever since. The feast/fast approach is his contribution to the fasting community, although its inception had nothing to do with the benefits of fasting.

Roman noticed that while he was getting a ton of benefit from cheat days in terms of fat loss and mental reprieve, the digestive aftermath wasn't pleasant. Many people report the same thing: if you cheat on Sunday, you may be paying for it on Monday in terms of intestinal distress. Not only are you likely to be in the bathroom more than you'd like, but also eating will feel like a chore.

As you can imagine, after a night of eating pasta, ice cream, brownies, and steak (yes, all at once), the last thing anyone wants to do first thing in the morning is eat. Eventually, Roman discarded the bodybuilding rule to eat a big breakfast, and he started pushing his first meal of the day back by a few hours . . . then a few more. Ultimately, he stopped eating altogether on the day following his cheat.

The results were impressive: Increased fat loss. More leanness. And better muscle definition. And, of course, a much happier tummy.

WHY IT WORKS

It almost seems too good to be true: trade one day of gluttony for one day without food and be better than where you started. Researching this concept has led us to stumble across a few different reasons why the feast/fast model works so well; some have to do with fasting, obviously, but some benefits are a direct result of cheating.

Like any style of fasting, removing food for an extended period of time can lead to fat loss because it often leads to lower caloric intake. Pretty simple. However, the reason this works well is because it's coming on the heels of a cheat day.

Remember, dieting causes leptin levels to drop, which slows down fat loss; strategically *overfeeding* boosts leptin levels back up, increasing the rate of fat loss. Putting a fast day after a cheat day, therefore, does two things:

1. Prevents any fat gain from the caloric spillover of eating, oh, we dunno, 14,000 calories worth of ice cream* by creating an immediate deficit

2. Prevents stagnated fat loss, allowing the hormonal benefit from the fast to proceed uninterrupted

More than anything, though, this is just a practical approach created to alleviate discomfort.

While the feast/fast model is undoubtedly a potent fat-loss technique, it's not a perfect system. The main drawback is that you're really looking at a thirty-two- to forty-hour fasting period. If your last meal on your cheat day is before bed (say, ten P.M.) on Sunday, and you don't eat at all on Monday, your first meal is breakfast Tuesday. And if you want to stick with your 16/8 schedule (which we recommend), that meal may not be until one P.M.

As you can probably guess, this has proven to be challenging for a number of people. That said, we believe that with some practice, just about anyone can abstain from food for an extended period of time with very little discomfort. Remember, when you fast, you're training decreased frequency of ghrelin secretion, meaning you control hunger, instead of it controlling you.

Still, for a lot of people, the idea of going without food for up to a day and a half is a bleak proposition. If you fall into this category, we're going to let you keep the training wheels on for a few weeks. So instead of the full-day fast, you can have a small dinner (up to 400 calories) on Monday night to take the edge off the hunger. This won't detract from any of the hormonal benefits (you still fast), but it does add some calories where there weren't any before. While this won't stop fat loss, it might slow the speed at which you can change your body.

---

* It *is* possible to eat 14,000 calories' worth of ice cream, by the way, and Roman has done it—twice. There is a monstrosity known as a Vermonster, a Ben & Jerry's confection made of twenty scoops of ice cream topped with four bananas, three chocolate chip cookies, a brownie, several ladles of hot fudge, and a mishmash of other toppings. Designed as a shared dessert suitable for feeding every attendee at a child's birthday party, the Vermonster is also considered an eating challenge. Very few people attempt to take the Vermonster down on their own, and fewer still accomplish it. Roman has attempted this twice, with one failure and one success to his credit. The success was documented in Tim Ferriss's bestseller *The 4-Hour Chef,* in which Roman is featured. Both Roman and Ferriss take their cheat days very seriously.

SCHEDULING YOUR FEAST/FAST

In the schedule we've provided you, cheat days fall on a Sunday with a full fast day following on Monday. This is not set in stone; you can really have your cheat day whenever you want—as long as you are able to follow it up with a fast. That said, understand that we've designed the entire workout and diet plan for convenience. So if you move your cheat day—and assuming you'll follow the plan and do a full fast after the cheat—then you need to realize that you will need to shift all the training days to correctly align with your workout days. We've provided a schedule to make this a thoughtless process.

While we're not going to give you a hard-and-fast rule for this, we strongly recommend scheduling your cheat day on Sunday (instead of Friday or Saturday) for three reasons.

1. **The NFL: We have anecdotal evidence showing that cheat days are more effective when they coincide with watching football.***

2. **The social aspect: For most of us, Sundays are lazy days—the days we don't have much scheduled to keep us busy and we get to spend time with our families and friends to just kick it.**** Given that cheat days allow for a diet that is more adaptable to socially friendly eating, we've found that Sundays make for the most logical and acceptable choice. Whether you're fifteen or fifty, it's hard to beat Sunday brunch with your family. So go enjoy some pancakes, all right?

3. **Practicality and staying occupied: Because you'll be fasting for a full thirty-six hours following the cheat day, it's best to arrange things so that your fast falls on a day when you're busy.** As the old saying goes, idle hands are the devil's playthings. In other words, if you are fasting on a day during which you're sitting at home doing nothing, like a Sunday, you're going to hear the Siren's call of food beckoning you from the kitchen a lot more frequently.

The busier you are, the easier it is to fast. By planning your fast on a workday, you create a situation where you're busy throughout the day, making adherence to the entire fast an easier process. For this reason, Monday makes the best fit for your full fast day, as it's generally the busiest day of the week. Trust us when we say that doing a fast day on a Sunday sucks.

Again, you can choose your own feast and fast days to fit your schedule. Just make sure that you reorganize the workout and fasting schedules accordingly. For example, if you want to cheat on Friday and make Saturday your fast day, don't randomly schedule your workouts to fall on Saturday. Instead, do the same training plan that we have scheduled

---

* Roman swears this is true. He also feels that the ability to console himself with food when the Jets lose is incredibly helpful. Or, as he puts it, "Scheduled properly, cheat days can make life as a Jets fan a little more bearable."

** People don't really say *kick it* anymore, which is regrettable. We're bringing it back. #alphastatus.

on cheat day, and do that on Friday. And then follow up with the training and fasting protocol on Saturday. The entire schedule has a rhyme and a reason. So maintain the diet and training pairings, and you'll be fine.

ADAPT: THE DIET

Determine Your Daily Caloric Intake During Adapt

Before you have your first cheat day, though, you once again need to determine your maintenance calories. This is done in precisely the same manner as in Prime, but *do not* use the same numbers. Your body will have undergone some radical changes in that four-week phase; at the very least, you'll have lost fat, which may put you into a different category of body fat. It's equally possible that you will have gained some muscle. In either case, your maintenance calories are going to be affected, and in order to make the best possible use of the program, you need to have the most accurate and current information. Therefore, before you set your goals for Adapt, please check your weight and get your body fat retested, and from there determine your *new* maintenance calories.

Done? Great. Let's move on to your daily calories. For Adapt, you're going to be eating below maintenance calories on both workout and non-workout days.

★ **To determine your calories for workout days, subtract 200 from your maintenance calories.**

★ **To determine your calories for non-workout days, subtract 600.**

You'll notice that you're eating a bit less on non-workout days in Adapt than you did in Prime; the reason is leptin. As mentioned, cheat days work because they serve to increase leptin; however, leptin levels only need a bump if they fall in response to a caloric deficit. To create the greatest possible effect, you'll eat a bit less during the week, but you'll *more* than make up for it with your cheat day.

MACRONUTRIENT BREAKDOWN

Protein

Once again, protein consumption is determined by your lean body mass, but it is higher during this phase.

Protein intake will be set as follows:

★ **Workout days:** 1 gram of protein per pound of LBM

★ **Non-workout days:** 0.8 grams of protein per pound of LBM

Carbs

★ **Workout days:** 0.75 grams per pound of LBM

★ **Non-workout days:** 0.3 grams per pound of LBM

Fat

At this point, you know your maintenance calories and have subtracted both the caloric values of your protein and carb intake. Now, you still have a balance of a few hundred calories; these will come from fat—and yes, that generally equates to a lot of fat. But as you know by now, if you're getting healthy fats, you're taking another step on the path toward hormonal optimization.

Now, as fat has 9 calories per gram, take your remaining balance of calories and divide by 9. The result is how many grams of fat you'll eat.

THE ALPHA EATING EQUATION: ADAPT

Workout Days

Going through the steps, it would look like this:

1. **Using the information in the chart on page 169, figure out how many calories you need in order to maintain your body weight.**

2. **Subtract 200 from that number.** Now we've got your calories for workout days.

3. **Multiply your lean body mass by 1.** This number represents how much protein you should eat.

4. **Multiply your lean body mass by 0.75.** This number represents how many carbs you should eat.

5. **Take your total grams of protein and your total grams of carbs, and add them together.**

6. **Multiply that number by 4.** This gives you the total number of calories from protein and carbs.

7. **Subtract this number from your calories for workout days.** This number is how many calories from fat you need.

8. **Divide this number by 9.** This is how many grams of fat you need.

Non-Workout Days

We repeat the same process for non-workout days:

1. **Using the information in the chart on page 169, figure out how many calories you need in order to maintain your body weight.**

2. **Subtract 600 from that number.** Now we've got your calories for non-workout days.

3. **Multiply your lean body mass by 0.8.** This number represents how much protein you should eat.

4. **Multiply your lean body mass by 0.3.** This number represents how many carbs you should eat.

5. **Take your total grams of protein and your total grams of carbs, and add them together.**

6. **Multiply that number by 4.** This gives you the total number of calories from protein and carbs.

7. **Subtract this number from your calories for non-workout days.** This number is how many calories from fat you need.

8. **Divide this number by 9.** This is how many grams of fat you need.

Now here's what it looks like in terms of food. Again, we provide examples of Roman and our fictional character, Steve. As you'll see, there is no shortage of good options.

With all of that covered, let's move on to the workouts for Phase II.

ROMAN: Phase II Meal Plan for Workout Days	Protein (grams)	Carbs (grams)	Fats (grams)	Calories
Contents				
First Solid Meal P+F Eye of round steak cooked in organic butter, 3 eggs, 2 slices tomato, 2 slices bacon, chopped and grilled zucchini with coconut oil	64	0	86	1030
Para-Workout Beverage P+C Workout Beverage—3 scoops BioTrust Low-Carb mixed with 12 oz fat-free milk. Consume ⅔ of this drink during the second half of your workout. Finish immediately upon completion.	50	30	5	365
Dinner Meal P+C+F Wild meat (bison, ostrich, venison, etc.) cooked in coconut oil, 2 cups cooked sticky rice, grilled onions and mushrooms in butter, 1 serving strawberries, free veggies	65	105	86	1454
Daily Totals	**179**	**135**	**177**	**2849**

ROMAN: Phase II Meal Plan for Non-Workout Days	Protein (grams)	Carbs (grams)	Fats (grams)	Calories
Contents				
First Solid Meal P+F Grilled chicken breast, ½ avocado, 3 eggs fried in coconut oil, chopped cucumber with salt and pepper	46	0	49	625
Midday Meal P+C+F Leg of lamb, 1 grilled eggplant, 1 cup cottage cheese, 4 tbsp almond butter, 1 cup mixed berries	46	35	50	774
Dinner Meal P+C+F Grilled shrimp and scallops with flank steak, 3 servings purple potatoes, roasted asparagus and cauliflower	51	100	50	1054
Daily Totals	**143**	**153**	**181**	**2453**

STEVE: Phase II Meal Plan for Workout Days				
Contents	Protein (grams)	Carbs (grams)	Fats (grams)	Calories
First Solid Meal P+F Small eye of round steak cooked in organic butter, 1 egg, 2 slices tomato, 2 slices bacon, chopped and grilled zucchini	55	0	48	652
Para-Workout Beverage P+C Workout Beverage—3 scoops BioTrust Low-Carb mixed with 12 oz fat-free milk. Consume ⅔ of this drink during the second half of your workout. Finish immediately upon completion.	50	30	5	365
Dinner Meal P+C+F Wild meat (bison, ostrich, venison, etc.) cooked in coconut oil, 2 cups cooked sticky rice, grilled onions and mushrooms in ½ serving butter, ½ cup strawberries, free veggies	55	90	49	1021
Daily Totals	**160**	**120**	**102**	**2038**

STEVE: Phase II Meal Plan for Non-Workout Days				
Contents	Protein (grams)	Carbs (grams)	Fats (grams)	Calories
First Solid Meal P+F Grilled chicken breast, ½ avocado, 1 egg fried in coconut oil, chopped cucumber with salt and pepper	43	0	24	388
Midday Meal P+C+F Leg of lamb, 1 grilled eggplant, 1 cup cottage cheese, 4 tbsp almond butter, 1 cup mixed berries	43	35	24	528
Dinner Meal P+C+F Grilled shrimp and scallops with flank steak, 2 servings purple potatoes, roasted asparagus and cauliflower	43	85	24	728
Daily Totals	**129**	**148**	**104**	**1644**

THE TRAINING

What Is Training Density?

Before we can talk about adding density training to your program, it's probably best to define the concept so you can understand why it's so effective. To compute your training density, you'll look at two very specific factors of training: volume and duration.

Volume: Your total workload—that is, how many total sets and reps you perform in a given workout

Duration: The length of time your workout lasts

By looking at these two things, we arrive at your training density, which is the measure of how much work you do (volume) in a given time period (duration).

Basic Methods for Increasing Training Density

For the most part, there are two simple and relatively well-known ways to increase training density. Both have been used effectively in the past.

Method 1—Subtract Time from the Duration
As an example, if you're doing 10 sets of 10 reps on the bench press, you're doing 100 total reps. Let's say this normally takes you 40 minutes; if we tell you that you must complete that workout in 30 minutes, then that will call for a drastic increase in training density—we're asking you to complete an identical amount of work in 25 percent less time.

Method 2—Add More Volume Within the Same Duration
Staying with that same example, you have another option. Keep the duration static at 40 minutes and simply add more sets within that time period. Rather than just doing 10 sets, you'd aim to complete as many sets as possible. You might wind up with 12 or even 15 sets. (This style of training is commonly known as *escalating* density training, or EDT. Charles Staley created it in 2001, and it has helped thousands of people gain muscle and lose fat since then. We've built on previously existing density protocols like EDT to make them even more effective.)

With both of these methods, you would have to increase training speed and decrease rest periods in order to fulfill the demands placed upon you by the new workout parameters.

Speaking generally, trainees seeking to increase density focus on one of the above. It comes down to either doing the same amount of work in less time or doing more work in the same amount of time. In the most extreme cases, a trainee in extremely good condition could potentially end up doing more work in less time and see phenomenal results.

Keeping in mind that increasing training density essentially increasing the amount of work you're doing in a given time frame, it stands to reason that over time you will also increase your ability to *do work* over any time period.

We call this your work capacity, and this determines how much you can realistically accomplish in the gym. Performing density-based training in any form increases your overall strength endurance and work capacity, and burns a huge amount of calories.

All of those things mean that not only is this great for fat loss, but increasing work capacity and strength endurance also has implications for increasing the rate of muscle hypertrophy. Translation: it becomes *a lot* easier to build muscle. And for most guys, that's usually the biggest hurdle. Well, this is your solution.

That alone would make it a good fat-burning protocol. But that's not enough for us. We developed a density-based protocol that takes fat burning to a whole other level.

In traditional density workouts, you simply seek to exceed the number of reps for each exercise on subsequent workouts. In that system, you're gauging progress from session to session. That's good, but we've found a way to add a dash of Alpha to density training. In Alpha density training, you see progress *during* the workout. In addition to performing more reps during the second set, you'll also be increasing the weight.

All told, the Alpha density workout consists of three circuits: A, B, and C. Each of these should be performed for the prescribed length of time and then repeated. In the case of circuits A and B, the weight should be increased prior to repeating the circuit. Circuit C maintains the same weight.

Circuit A

Two compound movements (one upper-body, one lower-body) will be alternated for 5 minutes. Select a weight for each exercise that you can lift 8–12 times. The goal is to get as many reps as possible within the 5-minute time frame—so do *not* go to failure. Instead, perform only 4–6 reps for the lower-body exercise; then put the weight down and perform 4–6 reps for the upper-body exercise. Alternate back and forth until the 5 minutes are up.

After this circuit, rest 3–5 minutes. Then increase your weights by 5 to 10 percent and repeat the circuit for another 5 minutes. After that circuit, rest 5 more minutes and proceed to circuit B.

Circuit B

Three compound movements (two upper, one lower) will be cycled for 6 minutes. Select weights you can lift 10–15 times. The goal is to get as many reps as possible within the 6-minute time frame—so do *not* perform these exercises to failure. Instead, perform only 4–6 reps for the first exercise; then put the weight down and perform 4–6 reps for the next, and then finally 4–6 reps for the final exercise. Keep cycling through these three exercises for 6 minutes.

After this circuit, rest 3–5 minutes. Then increase your weight by 3 to 5 percent and repeat the circuit for another 6 minutes. After that circuit, rest 5 more minutes and proceed to circuit C.

Circuit C

Two isolation movements will be alternated for 4 minutes. Select weights you can lift 10–15 times. The goal is to get as many reps as possible within the 4-minute time frame—so do *not* take each exercise to failure. Instead, perform only 4–6 reps for the first exercise; then put the weight down and perform 4–6 reps for the next exercise. Keep cycling through these two exercises for 4 minutes.

After this circuit, rest 2 minutes and then repeat the circuit with the same weight.

Now, of course it's hard to believe that you'll be able to do more weight and more reps on the second circuit of each of these exercises—and, to be fair, you won't always be able to. However, very often you'll exceed your reps from the previous set, and you'll almost always beat the total reps from your previous workout. This is what makes our Alpha density protocol special and unique—we take advantage of the fact that you often get stronger *during* a workout, which allows for greater total results.

In addition to helping you burn tons of fat, density training will increase your work capacity and help you get stronger while you retain LBM. And, of course, it helps you produce testosterone and combat estrogen-related fat storage.

HOW TO SPOT AN ALPHA IN THE GYM: PART II

By now you should be familiar with the Javelin Press, but we're going to add two other movements that will continue your progression from Prime and be an integral part of your workouts for the rest of the program. The other two Alpha movements are: the Alpha Press and the Alpha Deadlift.

Alpha Press

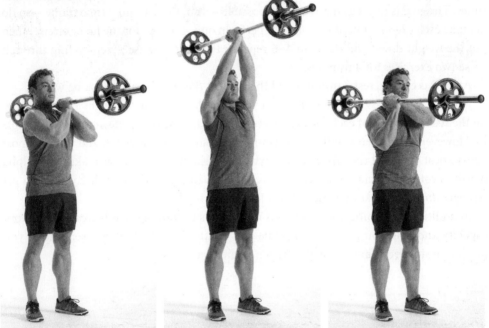

- Position a barbell lengthwise across one shoulder.

- Position your hands in the middle of the barbell, with one hand directly in front of the other.

- Press the barbell up, making sure to keep it level in the air.

- Press up and over your head; then lower down to the other shoulder.

As you perform this exercise, you should look like you're knighting yourself—touching first one shoulder, then the other. Change the position of your hands with each set (first left hand in front, then right hand in front, and so on).

Alpha Deadlift

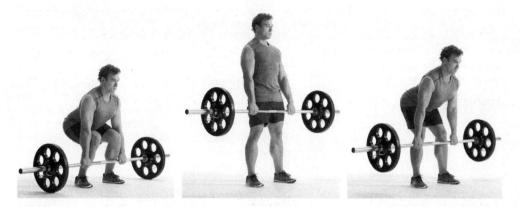

Up

● Grab a barbell in a double overhand grip.

● Bend your knees, squatting about two-thirds of the way down.

● Straighten your back and retract your shoulder blades.

● Initiate the lift by driving your heels into the ground and pulling *back* while straightening your hips.

● Lock out at the top of the movement with a hard squeeze of the glutes.

Down

● Bend your knees slightly and begin pushing your hips back.

● Lower the barbell toward the floor without bending your knees further.

● Push your hips back while maintaining tension in the hamstrings and keeping your back straight.

● Continue until the barbell touches the floor.

Both these exercises will feel harder and different than anything you've ever done before. Sure, you might get some stares in the gym, but they will turn into looks of jealousy when your body changes at a pace that seems almost unrealistic. And when that happens, you'll just nod at the other Alphas in the gym and do your best to spread the word. After all, sharing your knowledge is part of earning your Alpha status.

PHASE II WORKOUTS

Adapt Training Schedule							
	Monday	Tuesday	Wednesday	Thursday	Friday	Saturday	Sunday
Week 1 Training	Workout 1	Workout 2	OFF	Workout 3	OFF	OFF	Workout 4
Week 1 Nutrition	16/8	16/8	16/8	16/8	16/8	16/8	CHEAT DAY
Week 2 Training	Cardio	Workout 2	Workout 4	OFF	Workout 1	OFF	Workout 3
Week 2 Nutrition	FULL FAST	16/8	16/8	16/8	16/8	16/18	CHEAT DAY
Week 3 Training	Cardio	Workout 4	OFF	Workout 3	Workout 1	OFF	Workout 2
Week 3 Nutrition	FULL FAST	16/8	16/8	16/8	16/8	16/18	CHEAT DAY
Week 4 Training	Cardio	Workout 4	Workout 1	OFF	Workout 3	Workout 2	OFF
Week 4 Nutrition	FULL FAST	16/8	16/8	16/8	16/8	16/18	16/18

PHASE II, WORKOUT 1

A1 **Barbell Back Squat**
4–6 reps

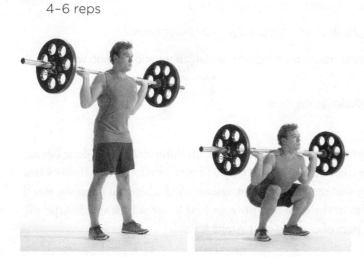

● Hold a barbell across your upper back with an overhand grip and your feet shoulder-width apart.

● Keeping your lower back arched, lower your body as deep as you can by pushing your hips back and bending your knees.

● Pause, then reverse the movement back to the starting position.

A2 Bent-Over Row
4-6 reps

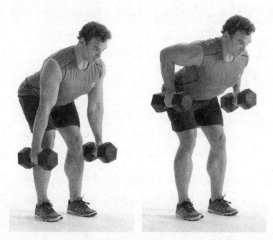

◗ Weight selection: pick a weight you could lift 8–12 times.

Alternate A1 and A2 for 5 minutes. The goal is to get as many reps as possible. After this circuit, rest 3–5 minutes. Then increase your weights by 5 to 10 percent and repeat the circuit for another 5 minutes. After the second time through, rest another 5 minutes and proceed to workout set B.

B1 Dumbbell Reverse Lunge
4-6 reps

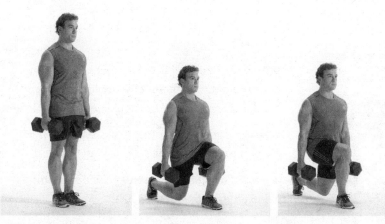

◗ Grab a pair of dumbbells and hold them at arm's length next to your sides, your palms facing each other.

◗ Step backward with your left leg.

◗ Lower your body into a lunge until your front leg is bent 90 degrees. Pause, then return to the starting position.

◗ Do all your reps and then repeat with your other leg.

B2 Dumbbell Upright Row
4–6 reps

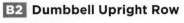

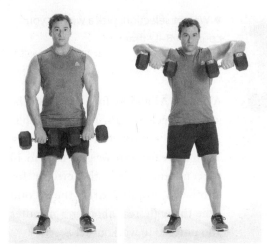

◗ Grab a pair of dumbbells with an overhand grip, and hold the weights in front of your thighs with your palms facing your body.

◗ Keeping the weights as close to your body as possible, pull the dumbbells up toward your chest. Your elbows should remain flared out during the movement.

◗ When the dumbbells are at your chest level (and not your chin), pause for 1 to 2 seconds, and then lower them back to the starting position.

B3 Flat Chest Press
4–6 reps

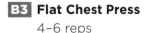

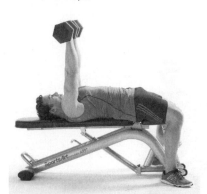

◗ Grab a pair of dumbbells and lie faceup on a flat bench.

◗ Hold the dumbbells above your chest with your arms straight. The dumbbells should be nearly touching, and your palms should be facing your feet.

◗ Keeping your elbows tucked close to your body, lower the weights to the sides of your chest.

◗ Weight selection: pick a weight you could lift 12–15 times.

Cycle through B1, B2, and B3 for 6 minutes. The goal is to get as many reps as possible. After this circuit, rest 3–5 minutes. Then increase your weights by 3 to 5 percent and repeat the circuit for another 6 minutes. After the second time through, rest another 5 minutes and proceed to workout set C.

C1 Dumbbell Biceps Curl
4–6 reps

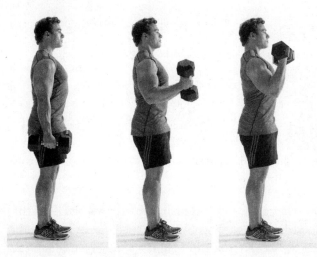

♦ Grab a pair of dumbbells and let them hang at arm's length next to your sides with your palms facing each other.

♦ Without moving your upper arms, bend your elbows and curl the dumbbells as close to your shoulders as you can.

♦ Pause, then lower the weights back to the starting position.

C2 Lateral Raise
4–6 reps

♦ Weight selection: pick a weight you could lift 8–12 times.

Alternate C1 and C2 for 4 minutes. The goal is to get as many reps as possible. After this circuit, rest 2 minutes and then repeat the circuit with the same weight.

PHASE II, WORKOUT 2

A1 **Alpha Deadlift**
   4–6 reps

A2 **Alpha Press**
   4–6 reps

◗ Weight selection: pick a weight you could lift 8–12 times.

Alternate A1 and A2 for 5 minutes. The goal is to get as many reps as possible. After this circuit, rest 3–5 minutes. Then increase your weights by 5 to 10 percent and repeat the circuit for another 5 minutes. After the second time through, rest another 5 minutes and proceed to workout set B.

B1 **Pull-Up or Lat Pull-Down**
   4–6 reps

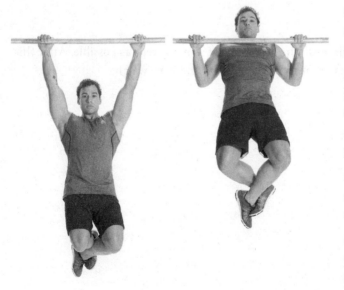

◗ Grab a chin-up bar with a shoulder-width overhand grip.

◗ Hang at arm's length and pull your shoulder blades down and back so that your shoulders are as far from your ears as possible.

◗ Pull your chest to the bar as you squeeze your shoulder blades together.

◗ Pause, and then lower your body back to a dead hang.

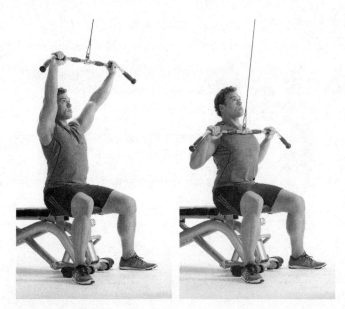

● Sit at a lat pull-down station and grab the bar with an overhand grip that's just beyond shoulder-width. Your arms should be completely straight and your torso upright.

● Pull your shoulder blades down and back, and bring the bar to your chest.

● Pause, then return to the starting position.

 Goblet Squat
4–6 reps

B3 **Push-Up**
4–6 reps

● Weight selection: pick a weight you could lift 12–15 times.

Cycle through B1, B2, and B3 for 6 minutes. The goal is to get as many reps as possible. After this circuit, rest 3–5 minutes. Then increase your weights by 3 to 5 percent and repeat the circuit for another 6 minutes. After the second time through, rest another 5 minutes and proceed to workout set C.

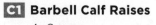 C1 Barbell Calf Raises
4–6 reps

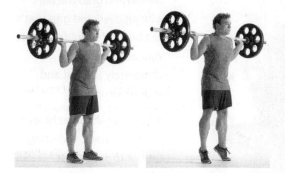

◗ Hold a barbell across your upper back with an overhand grip and your feet shoulder-width apart.

◗ Then, keeping your abs tight, lift your heels as high as you can.

◗ Pause, then lower and repeat.

C2 Dumbbell Fly
4–6 reps

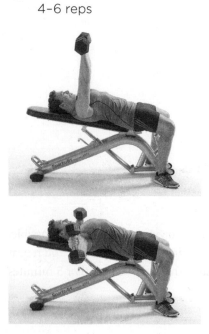

◗ Grab a pair of dumbbells and lie on your back on an inclined bench.

◗ Raise your arms straight above your chest with your palms facing forward and your elbows slightly bent.

◗ Slowly lower the dumbbells in an arc down and away from your body.

◗ Once the dumbbells are almost in line with your chest—but above it—reverse the movement back to the starting position, making sure you squeeze the muscles in your chest at the top of the movement.

◗ Weight selection: pick a weight you could lift 8–12 times.

Alternate C1 and C2 for 4 minutes. The goal is to get as many reps as possible. After this circuit, rest 2 minutes and then repeat the circuit with the same weight.

PHASE II, WORKOUT 3

A1 Trap Bar Deadlift
4–6 reps

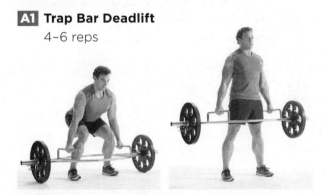

◗ Load a trap bar with weight, and stand between the trap bar handles with your feet about hip-width apart.

◗ Bend down, and grab the bar outside your knees. Your shoulders should be over the bar.

◗ Keeping your lower back in its natural arch, drive your heels into the floor and push your hips forward, lifting the bar until it's in front of your thighs.

◗ Lower the weight back to the starting position and repeat.

A2 Barbell High Pull
4–6 reps

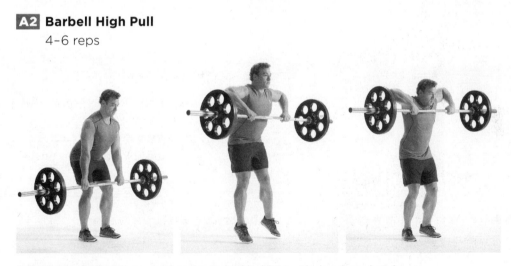

◗ Grab a barbell with an overhand grip and hold it just below knee height.

◗ Explosively pull the barbell upward, rise onto your toes, and bend your elbows as you bring the weight up to shoulder height. Return to the starting position.

◗ Weight selection: pick a weight you could lift 8–12 times.

Alternate A1 and A2 for 5 minutes. The goal is to get as many reps as possible. After this circuit, rest 3–5 minutes. Then increase your weights by 5 to 10 percent and repeat the circuit for another 5 minutes. After the second time through, rest another 5 minutes and proceed to workout set B.

B1 **Reverse Lunge**
4–6 reps

B2 **Face Pull**
4–6 reps

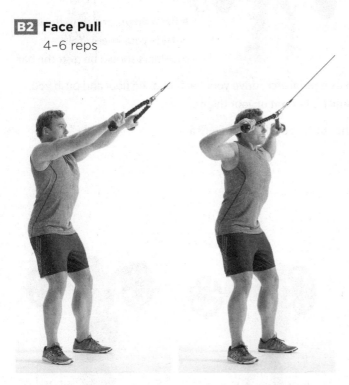

◗ Attach a rope to the high pulley of a cable station and grab an end with each hand so your palms face each other, thumbs toward you.

◗ Back a few steps away from the weight stack until your arms are straight in front of you and you feel tension in the cable.

◗ Pull the rope toward your eyes so your hands end up just outside your ears. You should be positioned in the classic bodybuilder's "double-biceps pose."

◗ Allow your arms to straighten out slowly in front of you and return to the start.

B3 **Barbell Push Press**
4–6 reps

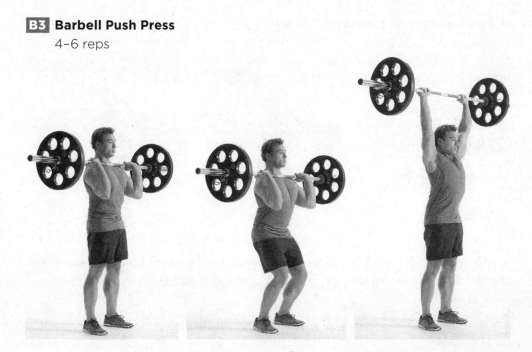

◆ Grab a barbell and hold it with a grip that's a little narrower than shoulder-width apart. Pull the barbell to just above your shoulders, and keep your elbows close to your body.

◆ Bend your knees and lower your body into a half squat.

◆ Press the weight overhead as you stand up tall and explode upward, pressing through your heels.

◆ Pause, then slowly lower the barbell back to the starting position.

◆ Weight selection: pick a weight you could lift 12–15 times.

Cycle through B1, B2, and B3 for 6 minutes. The goal is to get as many reps as possible. After this circuit, rest 3–5 minutes. Then increase your weights by 3 to 5 percent and repeat the circuit for another 6 minutes. After the second time through, rest another 5 minutes and proceed to workout set C.

C1 Dumbbell Rear Delt Fly
4-6 reps

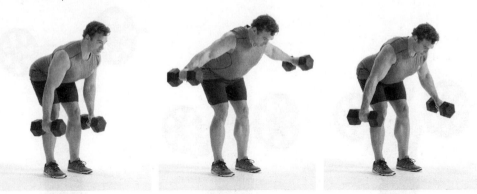

🔹 Grab a pair of dumbbells and bend forward at your hips until your back is nearly parallel to the floor. Your arms should hang straight down from your shoulders with your elbows slightly bent.

🔹 Hold your body still and raise your arms out to the sides until your hands are in line with your shoulders.

🔹 Pause, then return to the starting position.

C2 Barbell Reverse Curl
4-6 reps

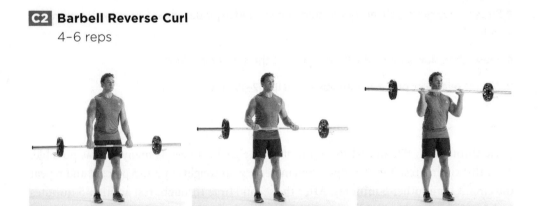

🔹 Weight selection: pick a weight you could lift 8–12 times.

Alternate C1 and C2 for 4 minutes. The goal is to get as many reps as possible. After this circuit, rest 2 minutes and then repeat the circuit with the same weight.

PHASE II, WORKOUT 4

A1 **Alpha Deadlift**
4–6 reps

A2 **Alpha Press**
4–6 reps

◆ Weight selection: pick a weight you could lift 8–12 times.

Alternate A1 and A2 for 5 minutes. The goal is to get as many reps as possible. After this circuit, rest 3–5 minutes. Then increase your weights by 5 to 10 percent and repeat the circuit for another 5 minutes. After the second time through, rest another 5 minutes and proceed to workout set B.

B1 **Inverted Row**
4–6 reps

B2 Hack Squat
4–6 reps

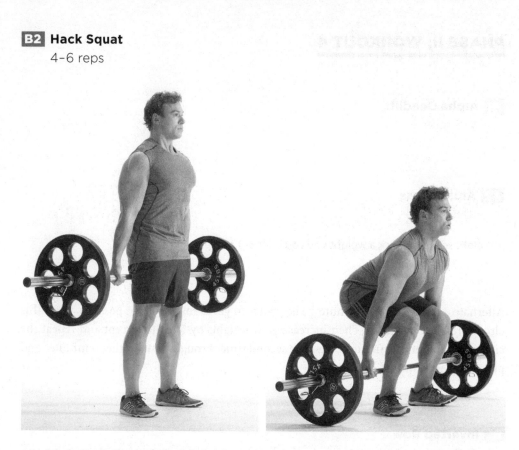

➧ Hold a barbell at arm's length behind your back, using a mixed grip (one hand overhand and one hand underhand). Stand with your feet shoulder-width apart.

➧ Keeping your lower back arched, lower your body as deep as you can. Initiate the movement by first pushing your hips back, then bend your knees.

➧ The tops of your thighs should be parallel to the floor or lower, and your torso should stay as upright as possible.

➧ Pause, then reverse the movement back to the starting position.

B3 Dumbbell Squeeze Press
4–6 reps

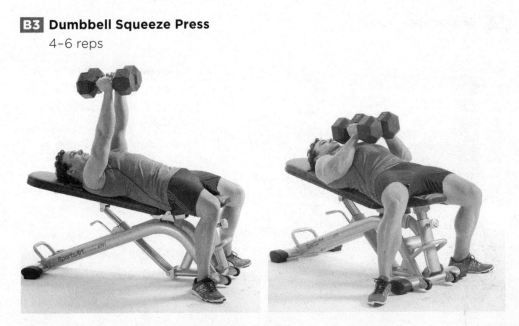

◆ Grab a pair of dumbbells and lie faceup on a slightly inclined bench.

◆ Hold the dumbbells above your chest with your arms straight.

◆ Then, press the dumbbells together as forcefully as possible, with your palms facing each other.

◆ Keeping your elbows tucked close to your body and the dumbbells in contact with one another, lower the weights to the sides of your chest.

◆ Pause, then press the dumbbells back above your chest.

◆ Weight selection: pick a weight you could lift 12–15 times.

Cycle through B1, B2, and B3 for 6 minutes. The goal is to get as many reps as possible. After this circuit, rest 3–5 minutes. Then increase your weights by 3 to 5 percent and repeat the circuit for another 6 minutes. After the second time through, rest another 5 minutes and proceed to workout set C.

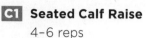

C1 Seated Calf Raise
4–6 reps

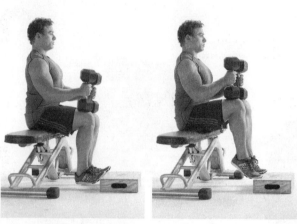

◗ Place a step in front of a bench, grab a pair of dumbbells, and sit down. Set the balls of both your feet on the step, and hold a dumbbell vertically on each knee.

◗ Lower both heels as far as you can without touching the floor.

◗ Push off the balls of your feet and lift your heels as high as you can.

C2 Dumbbell Shrugs
4–6 reps

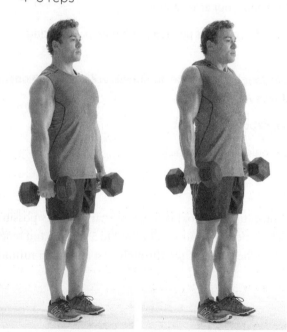

◗ Grab a pair of dumbbells and let them hang at arm's length with your palms facing each other.

◗ In one movement, explode upward and shrug your shoulders as high as you can, while keeping your arms straight.

◗ Weight selection: pick a weight you could lift 8–12 times.

Alternate C1 and C2 for 4 minutes. The goal is to get as many reps as possible. After this circuit, rest 2 minutes and then repeat the circuit with the same weight.

CHAPTER 11

Phase III: Surge

BREAKING THE MOLD

"It is not by muscle, speed, or physical dexterity that great things are achieved, but by reflection, force of character, and judgment."

—MARCUS TULLIUS CICERO

The old saying goes that the easiest way to look like you've added muscle is to lose fat. And when you think about it, the concept makes perfect sense. We all have muscle, but fat hides it. This is only true up to a certain point, though.

By now, you should have lost a significant amount of fat. Your clothes should look better, you should be able to see more of your body, and your muscles should be bigger and harder. But the truth is, although we've been targeting your hormones and increasing testosterone, we've yet to specifically focus on muscle growth, which should excite all of you. You've gained muscle already as a by-product of hormonal optimization, and now we're going to kick your body into hyperdrive so you can have bigger muscles and even less fat.

That's the point of Surge. This isn't about suddenly becoming big and bulky. Quite the opposite—this is where you get stronger while maintaining your lean body. We'll accomplish this by focusing on two new hormones: growth hormone (GH) and cortisol. Specifically, we'll be increasing your GH and decreasing your cortisol. When combined with your improved insulin sensitivity, raised testosterone, and decreased estrogen, you've created a hormonal environment that will actually allow you to build significant muscle without gaining fat.

THE METHOD BEHIND THE MUSCLE

Unlike metabolic resistance training—which essentially just focuses on exercise order and short rest periods—GH-based programs require us to take a more roundabout approach, as you'll learn in Surge. While GH training isn't perfect, if you're focusing on losing fat while gaining muscle, it's one of the best methods you can use. We've built your body up in a progressive way, so at this point, your body is primed for growth.

While almost any workout will increase GH, if you want to send GH production through the roof, you want to be looking at lactic acid.

Lactic Acid and Training

With regard to exercise specifically, lactic acid is a chemical waste by-product that is created during certain chemical reactions generated by resistance training. As lactic acid metabolites—a substance produced by the increased metabolism triggered by weight training—begin to flood the bloodstream, this increases the overall acidity (makes sense—it's called lactic *acid* after all) of the extracellular tissues, and nerve irritation occurs.

When your blood and nerves and other tissues are all acid-y, your body goes, "Dude, this sucks. I'm going to fix it." Basically, because the cycle of metabolic waste removal is breaking down, certain processes begin to regulate acidity.

Lactic Acid and Growth Hormone

In order to regulate acidity, your pituitary gland will begin to produce and secrete tremendous amounts of GH, which is the single most effective biological compound your body can produce to elicit fat loss and muscle gain.

Simply stated, training in a way that produces a lot of lactic acid—and thereby signals immense release of GH—is one of the single most effective ways to trigger simultaneous fat loss and muscle gain, especially if you're in a caloric deficit of any kind (as you will be on non-workout days).

As an added benefit, GH is specifically beneficial in that it can counteract the fat-storing effects of cortisol. You see, GH has an inverse relationship with cortisol—as GH goes up, cortisol goes down. And this combination is what will help you sleep better, provide an overall increase in feelings of wellness, and make it harder for your body to store belly fat.

The important thing to note is that lactic acid is produced predominantly during the concentric (or positive) phase of the movement. So when you're actually *lifting* the weight (think about squeezing a weight at the top of a biceps curl), you're producing a lot more lactic acid than when you're lowering it.

In order to maximize production of lactic acid, we simply modify our lifting speed to take the greatest advantage of that fact. With most training modalities, you're using a 2-0-2 cadence. This means that you're lifting the weight for two seconds, pausing for zero seconds at the top of the motion, and then lowering the weight for two seconds. In some cases, you'll use a 2-0-3 cadence, which is just a slower lowering phase.

In keeping with that line of thought, lactic acid training can, to some degree, be thought of as inverted tempo training. To that, we lift the weight over a period of four seconds (in most cases) and lower extremely fast in order to allow for nearly constant concentric tension and high levels of lactic acid production.

To give an example, if you were doing an overhead press, a single rep would appear like this:

Lift the weight over a period of 4 seconds

Lower the weight as quickly as possible in good form

Immediately begin lifting again

To reiterate, lifting in this way produces a tremendous amount of lactic acid, which in turn forces your body to produce exceptionally high amounts of GH, which is what will make the transformations during this third phase some of the most fun.

SURGE: THE DIET

Determine Your Daily Caloric Intake During Surge

Before you can do this, you once again need to determine your maintenance calories. This is done in precisely the same manner as in Prime and Adapt; again, your body will have undergone some radical changes and in order to make the best possible use of the program, you need to have the most accurate and current information. Therefore, before you can progress any farther, please check your weight and get your body fat retested, and from there determine your *new* maintenance calories.

Surge is the first time you'll be eating above maintenance calories. Because of the long period of deficit and the hormonal environment you've created, your body is prepared to grow. In this phase, we'll be taking in more calories and pairing the diet with a training modality specifically intended to increase GH—that, coupled with the volume, will lead to tremendous growth. So we hope you brought your appetite.

Specifically, you're going to be eating *above* maintenance calories on workout days and *below* maintenance calories on non-workout days.

★ **To determine your calories for workout days, add 400 to your maintenance calories.**

★ **To determine your calories for non-workout days, subtract 200.**

MACRONUTRIENT BREAKDOWN

Protein

Once again, protein is determined by your lean body mass, but it's higher during this phase. Protein intake will be set as follows:

★ **Workout days:** 1.5 grams of protein per pound of LBM

★ **Non-workout days:** 1.25 grams of protein per pound of LBM

Carbs

★ **Workout days:** 1 gram per pound of LBM

★ **Non-Workout days:** 0.5 grams per pound of LBM

Fat

At this point, you know your maintenance calories and have subtracted the caloric values of both your protein and carb intakes. Now, you still have a balance of a few hundred calories; these will come from fat—and yes, that generally equates to a lot of fat. But, as you know by now, if you're getting healthy fats, you're taking another step on the path toward hormonal optimization.

Now, as fat has 9 calories per gram, take your remaining balance of calories and divide by 9. The result is how many grams of fat you eat.

THE ALPHA EATING EQUATION: SURGE

Workout Days

Going through the steps, it would look like this:

1. **Using the information in the chart on page 169, figure out how many calories you need in order to maintain your body weight.**

2. **Add 400 to that number.** Now we've got your calories for workout days.

3. **Multiply your lean body mass by 1.5.** This number represents how much protein you should eat.

4. **Multiply your lean body mass by 1.25.** This number represents how many carbs you should eat.

5. **Take your total grams of protein and your total grams of carbs, and add them together.**

6. **Multiply that number by 4.** This gives you the total number of calories from protein and carbs.

7. **Subtract this number from your calories for workout days.** This number is how many calories from fat you need.

8. **Divide this number by 9.** This is how many grams of fat you need.

That's it—just eight simple steps, and you know exactly how many grams of carbs, fat, and protein you should be taking in.

Non-Workout Days

We repeat the same process for non-workout days:

1. **Using the information in the chart on page 169, figure out how many calories you need in order to maintain your body weight.**

2. **Subtract 200 from that number.** Now we've got your calories for non-workout days.

3. **Multiply your lean body mass by 1.25.** This number represents how much protein you should eat.

4. **Multiply your lean body mass by 0.5.** This number represents how many carbs you should eat.

5. **Take your total grams of protein and your total grams of carbs, and add them together.**

6. **Multiply that number by 4.** This gives you the total number of calories from protein and carbs.

7. **Subtract this number from your calories for non-workout days.** This number is how many calories from fat you need.

8. **Divide this number by 9.** This is how many grams of fat you need.

Let's take a look at Roman's and Steve's sample menus for Phase III:

ROMAN: Phase III Meal Plan for Workout Days				
Contents	**Protein** (grams)	**Carbs** (grams)	**Fats** (grams)	**Calories**
First Solid Meal P+F ½ rotisserie chicken; ½ avocado; chopped onion, mushroom, spinach, kale, all grilled in butter or coconut oil; 3 eggs	109	0	80	1156
Para-Workout Beverage P+C Workout Beverage—3 scoops BioTrust Low-Carb mixed with 12 oz fat-free milk. Consume ⅔ of this drink during the second half of your workout. Finish immediately upon completion.	50	30	5	365
Dinner Meal P+C+F Large trout, grilled Brussels sprouts in organic butter with roasted nuts and bacon, 4 servings baby potatoes roasted or boiled, topped with 2 servings olive oil / vinegar	110	194	79	1927
Daily Totals	**269**	**224**	**195**	**3700**

ROMAN: Phase III Meal Plan for Non-Workout Days				
Contents	**Protein** (grams)	**Carbs** (grams)	**Fats** (grams)	**Calories**
First Solid Meal P+F Extra-lean ground steak with spices, 2 servings olives, chopped pepper, 1 small can sardines in olive oil	59	0	62	794
Midday Meal P+C+F Large pork tenderloin; ½ sweet potato and organic butter; ½ cup strawberries blended with cocoa, ½ cup heavy cream, cinnamon, 2 cups spinach, and vanilla extract to taste	60	30	62	918
Dinner Meal P+C+F Frozen and cooked king crab; 3 strips bacon; 2 cups cooked quinoa with chopped mixed vegetables, sprinkle of pumpkin seeds	60	60	62	1038
Daily Totals	**179**	**90**	**186**	**2750**

STEVE: Phase III Meal Plan for Workout Days				
Contents	**Protein** (grams)	**Carbs** (grams)	**Fats** (grams)	**Calories**
First Solid Meal P+F ½ rotisserie chicken; chopped onion, mushroom, spinach, and kale, all grilled in butter or coconut oil; 1 egg	95	0	48	794
Para-Workout Beverage P+C Workout Beverage—3 scoops BioTrust Low-Carb mixed with 12 oz fat-free milk. Consume ⅔ of this drink during the second half of your workout. Finish immediately upon completion.	50	30	5	365
Dinner Meal P+C+F Large trout; grilled Brussels sprouts in organic butter with roasted nuts; 3 servings baby potatoes roasted or boiled, topped with 1 serving olive oil / vinegar	95	170	47	1483
Daily Totals	**240**	**200**	**100**	**2642**

STEVE: Phase III Meal Plan for Non-Workout Days				
Contents	**Protein** (grams)	**Carbs** (grams)	**Fats** (grams)	**Calories**
First Solid Meal P+F Extra-lean ground steak with spices, 1 serving olives, chopped pepper, 1 small can sardines in water	53	0	36	536
Midday Meal P+C+F Large pork tenderloin; ½ cup strawberries blended with cocoa, ½ cup heavy cream, cinnamon, 2 cups spinach, and vanilla extract to taste	53	20	36	616
Dinner Meal P+C+F Frozen and cooked king crab, 1 strip bacon, 2 cups cooked quinoa with chopped mixed vegetables	54	60	36	780
Daily Totals	**160**	**80**	**120**	**2040**

PHASE III WORKOUTS

Surge Training Schedule							
	Monday	Tuesday	Wednesday	Thursday	Friday	Saturday	Sunday
Week 1	Workout 1	Workout 2	OFF	Workout 3	OFF	Workout 4	OFF
Week 2	Workout 3	Workout 1	OFF	Workout 4	OFF	Workout 2	OFF
Week 3	Workout 4	Workout 3	OFF	Workout 2	OFF	Workout 1	OFF
Week 4	Workout 2	Workout 4	OFF	Workout 1	OFF	Workout 3	OFF

PHASE III, WORKOUT 1

A Squat (any variation)
20 reps

Note that this is *not* a lactic acid–based exercise. This is a 20-rep set done with a challenging weight at a normal tempo. After this set, rest 2–3 minutes and proceed to B.

B1 Chest Press
12 reps

B2 Barbell Bent-Over Row
10 reps

B3 Plank
Hold for 60 seconds

This circuit consists of two exercises performed lactic-acid style at a tempo of 1-0-4 for 10–12 reps each for 3 sets. Select a weight appropriate for each exercise (often, different weights each circuit). Tempo does not factor in for the plank. Simply hold for 60 seconds.

Perform exercises B1–B3 sequentially, resting 10–30 seconds between exercises. After B3, rest 90 seconds and repeat. After your last circuit, rest 2 minutes and proceed to workout set C.

C1 Lateral Raise
12 reps

C2 Romanian Dumbbell Deadlift
8 reps

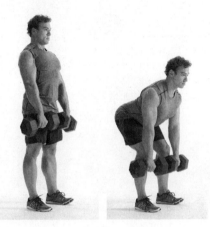

This circuit consists of two exercises performed at a tempo of 1-0-4 for 8–12 reps each, a total of 4 times. Select a weight appropriate for each exercise (often, different weights each circuit). Perform exercises C1–C2 sequentially, resting 10 seconds between exercises. After C2, rest 90 seconds and repeat. After your last set, rest 2 minutes and proceed to workout set D.

D Body-Weight Squat
25 reps

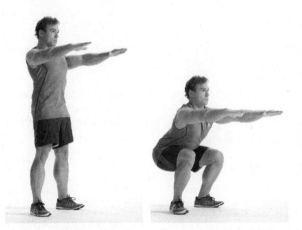

◗ Stand tall with your feet shoulder-width apart and place your arms forward, palms facing down.

◗ Lower your body as far as you can by pushing your hips back and bending your knees.

◗ Pause, then push yourself back to the starting position.

Again, this is *not* a lactic acid–based exercise. This is a 25-rep set done at a normal tempo with *only* your body weight.

PHASE III, WORKOUT 2

A Trap Bar Deadlifts from Deficit
20 reps

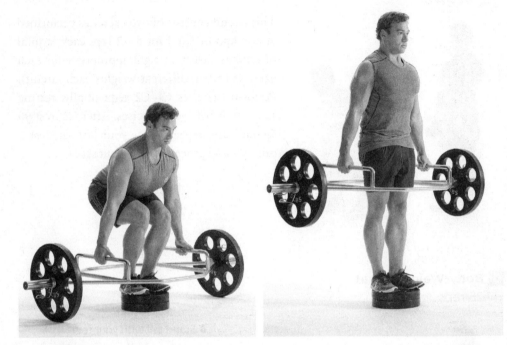

◆ Load a trap bar with weight, and stand on a short box or a weight plate between the trap bar handles with your feet about hip-width apart.

◆ Bend down, and grab the bar outside your knees. Your shoulders should be over the bar.

◆ Keeping your lower back in its natural arch, drive your heels into the floor and push your hips forward, lifting the bar until it's in front of your thighs.

◆ Lower the weight back to the starting position and repeat.

This is *not* a lactic acid–based exercise. This is a 20-rep set done with challenging weight at a normal tempo. After this set, rest 2–3 minutes and proceed to workout set B.

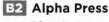
Pull-Up or Pull-Down
10 reps

May use assisted pull-ups or any variation of pull-downs, including resistance bands.

B2 Alpha Press
10 reps

B3 Feet-Elevated Plank
45 seconds

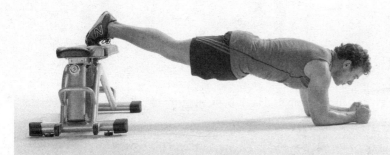

◆ Start to get in a push-up position, but bend your elbows and rest your weight on your forearms instead of on your hands. Then, place your feet on a bench. Your body should form a straight line from your shoulders to your ankles.

◆ Brace your core by contracting your abs as if you were about to be punched in the gut.

◆ Hold this position as directed.

These are *not* lactic acid–based exercises. Perform them at a normal tempo. Select a weight appropriate for each exercise (often, different weights each circuit). Tempo does not factor in for the plank. Simply hold for 60 seconds.

Perform exercises B1–B3 sequentially, resting 10–30 seconds between exercises. After B3, rest 60 seconds and repeat. After your last circuit, rest 2 minutes and proceed to workout set C.

C1 Push-Up
12 reps

C2 Barbell Biceps Curl
15 reps

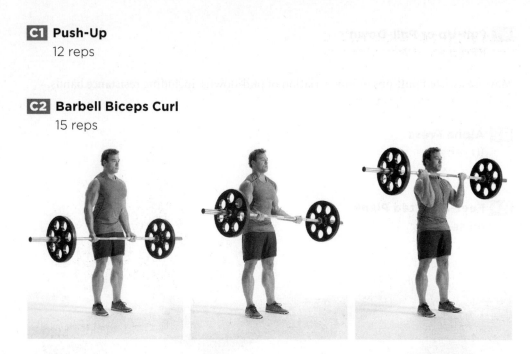

♦ Grab a barbell with an underhand grip and let it hang at arm's length with your palms facing forward.

♦ Without moving your upper arms, bend your elbows and curl the barbell as close to your shoulders as you can.

♦ Pause, then lower the barbell back to the starting position.

These two exercises are performed lactic-acid style at a tempo of 3-0-1 for 12–15 reps each, a total of 5 times. Select a weight appropriate for each exercise (often, different weights each circuit). Perform exercises C1–C2 sequentially, resting 10 seconds between exercises. After C2, rest 90 seconds and repeat. After your last set, rest 2 minutes and proceed to workout set D.

D Trap Bar Deadlifts from Deficit
25 reps

This is *not* a lactic acid–based exercise. This is a 25-rep set done with light weight. Use 20 to 30 percent of the weight you used for workout set A, and perform it at a steady tempo.

PHASE III, WORKOUT 3

A Rack Pull from the Knee
20 reps

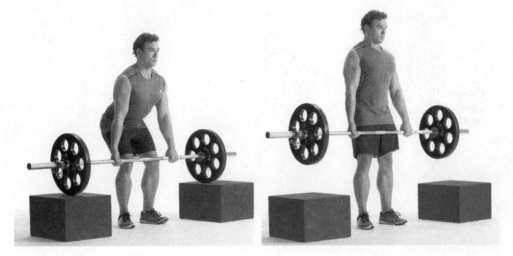

🔸 Set the pins on a lifting platform to a level that's just below knee-height when you're standing tall.

🔸 Load a barbell on the pins and grab the bar with an overhand grip

🔸 Bend at your hips and knees, and without allowing your lower back to round, stand up, thrust your hips forward, and squeeze your glutes.

🔸 Pause, then lower the bar back to the lifting platform while keeping it as close to your body as possible.

This is *not* a lactic acid–based exercise. This is a 20-rep set done with challenging weight at a steady tempo. After this set, rest 2–3 minutes and proceed to workout set B.

B1 High-Incline Dumbbell Bench Press
12 reps

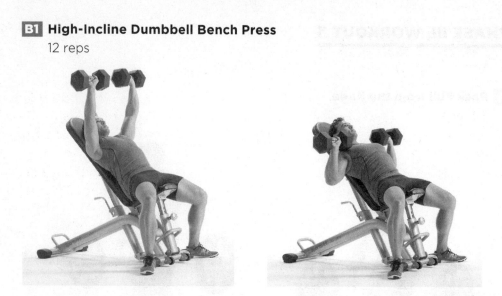

▶ Set an adjustable bench to an incline of 45 to 60 degrees.

▶ Grab a pair of dumbbells and lie faceup on the bench. Hold the dumbbells directly above your shoulders with your arms straight.

▶ Lower the dumbbells to the sides of your chest, pause, and then press the weights back above your chest.

B2 Seated Cable Row
10 reps

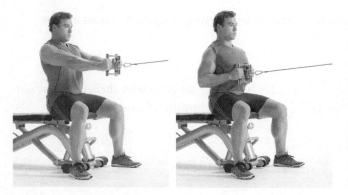

▶ Attach a straight bar or stirrup attachment to the cable machine and position your body (as seen) with your feet braced.

▶ Grab the attachment, bend your knees slightly, and sit up straight with your shoulders down and back.

▶ Without moving your torso, pull the bar or stirrup toward your upper abs. Pause, then return to the starting position.

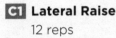 **Plank**
Hold for 60 seconds

This circuit consists of three exercises performed lactic-acid style at a tempo of 4-0-1 for 8–12 reps each, a total of 3 times. Select a weight appropriate for each exercise (often, different weights each circuit). Tempo does not factor in for the plank. Simply hold for 60 seconds.

Perform exercises B1–B3 sequentially, resting 10–30 seconds between exercises. After B3, rest 90 seconds and repeat. After your last circuit, rest 2 minutes and proceed to workout set C.

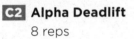 **Lateral Raise**
12 reps

C2 **Alpha Deadlift**
8 reps

This circuit consists of two exercises performed at a tempo of 4-0-1 for 8–12 reps each, a total of 4 times. Select a weight appropriate for each exercise (often, different weights each circuit). Perform exercises C1–C2 sequentially, resting 10 seconds between exercises. After C2, rest 90 seconds and repeat. After your last set, rest 2 minutes and proceed to workout set D.

D **Rack Pull from the Knee**
25 reps

This is *not* a lactic acid–based exercise. This is a 25-rep set done at a steady tempo. Use 20 to 30 percent of the weight you used for workout set A.

PHASE III, WORKOUT 4

A Alpha Deadlift
20 reps

This is *not* a lactic acid–based exercise. This is a 20-rep set done at a steady tempo with challenging weight. After this set, rest 2–3 minutes and proceed to workout set B.

B1 Bent-Over Row
10 reps

May use assisted pull-ups or any variation of pull-downs, including resistance bands.

B2 Low-Incline Dumbbell Bench Press
10 reps

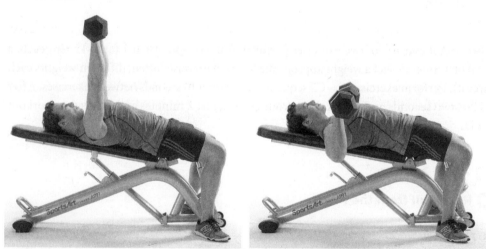

● Set an adjustable bench to an incline of 15 to 30 degrees.

● Grab a pair of dumbbells and lie faceup on the bench. Hold the dumbbells directly above your shoulders with your arms straight and your palms facing forward.

● Lower the dumbbells to the sides of your chest, pause, and then press the weights back above your chest.

Feet-Elevated Plank
45 seconds

Tempo does not factor in here, simply hold for 45 seconds.

This is *not* a lactic acid–based exercise. This circuit consists of three exercises performed 10 reps each at a steady tempo a total of 4 times. Select a weight appropriate for each exercise (often, different weights each circuit). Perform exercises B1–B3 sequentially, resting 10–30 seconds between exercises. After B3, rest 60 seconds and repeat. After your last circuit, rest 2 minutes and proceed to workout set C.

C1 **Dumbbell Rear Delt Fly**
12 reps

C2 **Body-Weight Glute Bridge**
15 reps

These two exercises are performed lactic-acid style at a tempo of 3-0-1 for 12–15 reps each, a total of 5 times. Select a weight appropriate for each exercise (often, different weights each circuit). Perform exercises C1–C2 sequentially, resting 10 seconds between exercises. After C2, rest 90 seconds and repeat. After your last set, rest 2 minutes and proceed to workout set D.

D **Alpha Deadlifts**
25 reps

This is *not* a lactic acid–based exercise. This is a 25-rep set done with light weight. Use 20 to 30 percent of the weight you used for workout set A.

CHAPTER 12

Phase IV: Complete

THE END OF THE BEGINNING

"A man who as a physical being is always turned toward the outside, thinking that his happiness lies outside him, finally turns inward and discovers that the source is within him."

—SÖREN KIERKEGAARD

Some fitness programs fizzle out. Others just end. We made it a point to make sure that when you finish this workout and diet, you'll feel complete. This isn't about reaching an end goal. This is more about *complete* satisfaction with the changes you hoped to make and the improvements you've always wanted.

Complete is a four-week phase designed to help you become the hero in your journey; it is the last aspect of engineering you into the Alpha you were meant to be, helping you polish off your physique so you look and feel better than ever.

In many ways, we consider Phase IV to be the all-star program. And since by now you know just how truly nerdy we are, you won't be at all surprised that we'll compare this phase to superheroes.

In comic books, superheroes often gather into groups or teams; from the X-Men to the Fantastic 4, the Justice League to the Avengers, heroes recognize that in order to save the world, you need various skill sets. In order to write compelling story lines, comic book authors realize that having superheroes work together in a way that allows their powers to complement one another creates a unit whose value is greater than the sum of its parts.

Well, in Phase IV, we want to recreate that with a comprehensive approach to all the phases you've already experienced.

In the previous phases, we've focused on specific hormones and the modality to address each: insulin and metabolic resistance training, testosterone and density training, GH and GH-surge training. All of these things helped you lose fat, build muscle, or gain strength. And sometimes you experienced multiple benefits at the same time as a result of hard training, improved diet, and better hormone functioning.

Now that we have developed each of those qualities, it's time to teach your body to develop them together. Just as any superhero team—or any team, for that matter—has to train together for a while in order to develop a rhythm and become effective together, so too must your training encompass all of the various qualities at once.

By working through Phase IV, you will finish the program with your insulin sensitivity as high as it was in Prime, your body as lean as you were in Adapt, and your muscles as strong as they were in Surge. In fact, you'll likely burn off any extra fat that you may have, increase muscle in some key areas, and even get a bit stronger.

In order to accomplish this, Complete combines one day of fat-loss training, one day of density-based training, one day of muscle building, and one day of strength work.

This phase lasts four weeks and, again, is intended to help you finalize your physique and set you up to dominate any program you decide to do after you achieve Alpha status.

COMPLETE: THE DIET

Determine Your Daily Caloric Intake During Complete

Before you can do this, you once again need to determine your maintenance calories. This is done in precisely the same manner as in Prime and Adapt and Surge. As always, before you go any farther, please check your weight and get your body fat retested, and from there determine your new maintenance calories.

Done? Great. Let's move on to your daily calories. As with Surge, you're going to be eating *above* maintenance calories on workout days and below maintenance calories on non-workout days during Complete.

★ **To determine your calories for workout days, add 300 to your daily calories.**

★ **To determine your calories for non-workout days, subtract 400.**

In this phase, we are decreasing the surplus on workout days, and increasing the deficit on non-workout days. In this phase, we'll be taking in fewer calories and pairing the diet with a training modality specifically intended to increase GH—that, coupled with the volume, will lead to tremendous growth.

MACRONUTRIENT BREAKDOWN

Protein

Once again, protein consumption is determined by your lean body mass, but it's higher during this phase. Protein intake will be set as follows:

★ **Workout days:** 1.5 grams of protein per pound of LBM

★ **Non-workout days:** 1 gram of protein per pound of LBM

Carbs

★ **Workout days:** 1 gram of carbs per pound of LBM

★ **Non-workout days:** 0.25 grams of carbs per pound of LBM

Fat

At this point, you know your maintenance calories and have subtracted the caloric values of both your protein and carb intakes. Now, you still have a balance of a few hundred calories; these will come from fat—and yes, that generally equates to a lot of fat. But, as you know by now, if you're getting healthy fats, you're taking another step on the path toward hormonal optimization.

Now, as fat has 9 calories per gram, take your remaining balance of calories and divide by 9. The result is how many grams of fat you'll eat.

THE ALPHA EATING EQUATION: COMPLETE

Workout Days

Going through the steps, it would look like this:

1. **Using the information in the chart on page 169, figure out how many calories you need in order to maintain your body weight.**

2. **Add 300 to that number.** Now we've got your calories for workout days.

3. **Multiply your lean body mass by 1.5.** This number represents how much protein you should eat.

4. **Multiply your lean body mass by 1.** This number represents how many carbs you should eat.

5. **Take your total grams of protein and your total grams of carbs, and add them together.**

6. **Multiply that number by 4.** This gives you the total number of calories from protein and carbs.

7. **Subtract this number from your calories for workout days.** This number is how many calories from fat you need.

8. **Divide this number by 9.** This is how many grams of fat you need.

Non-Workout Days

1. **Using the information in the chart on page 169, figure out how many calories you need in order to maintain your body weight.**

2. **Subtract 400 from that number.** Now we've got your calories for non-workout days.

3. **Multiply your lean body mass by 1.** This number represents how much protein you should eat.

4. **Multiply your lean body mass by 0.25.** This number represents how many carbs you should eat.

5. **Take your total grams of protein and your total grams of carbs, and add them together.**

6. **Multiply that number by 4.** This gives you the total number of calories from protein and carbs.

7. **Subtract this number from your calories for non-workout days.** This number is how many calories from fat you need.

8. **Divide this number by 9.** This is how many grams of fat you need.

Steve: 200 Pounds
20% Body Fat LBM: 160 Baseline Calories = 2,240
Workout Days
Calories = 2,240 + 300 = 2,540 Protein = 160 x 1.5 = 240 grams Carbs = 160 x 1 = 160 grams
Carbs + Protein = 400 Grams x 4 = 1,600 calories 2,540 - 1,600 = 940 calories Fat = 940/9 = 104 grams of fat
Non-Workout Days
Calories = 2,240 – 400 = 1,840 Protein = 160 grams Carbs = 40 grams
Carbs + Protein = 200 grams x 4 = 800 calories 1,840 – 800 = 1,040 calories Fat = 1,040/9 = 116 grams of fat

See how Roman adjusts his diet for these caloric needs and how Steve's diet might look too.

ROMAN: Phase IV Meal Plan for Workout Days				
Contents	**Protein** (grams)	**Carbs** (grams)	**Fats** (grams)	**Calories**
First Solid Meal P+F Gourmet omelet of 8 whole eggs, 1 tbsp coconut oil, spinach, mixed veggies, low-carb Parmesan, cheddar, 3 turkey sausages, and low-carb hot sauce	109	0	84	1192
Para-Workout Beverage P+C Workout Beverage—3 scoops BioTrust Low-Carb mixed with 12 oz fat-free milk. Consume ⅔ of this drink during the second half of your workout. Finish immediately upon completion.	50	30	5	365
Dinner Meal P+C+F 1 large filet mignon, 3 slices peameal bacon, 2 tbsp organic butter, tossed tomato, cabbage, cucumber, radish, ½ cup sauerkraut, 3 large baked potatoes with salt and butter	110	149	84	1792
Daily Totals	**269**	**179**	**173**	**3349**

ROMAN: Phase IV Meal Plan for Non-Workout Days				
Contents	**Protein** (grams)	**Carbs** (grams)	**Fats** (grams)	**Calories**
First Solid Meal P+F 4 large chicken thighs, seaweed salad with lemon and herbs, macadamia oil, ½ avocado	59	0	65	821
Midday Meal P+C+F Large steak of kangaroo or boar, onions fried in organic butter, kale and baby greens salad with tomato, ½ cup chopped bacon, and 1 tbsp macadamia nut oil	60	0	65	825
Dinner Meal P+C+F Large turkey breast, 2 servings organic pesto, 1 cup jasmine rice fried in organic butter with chopped broccoli and choice of spices, topped with 1 serving roasted nuts	60	45	65	1005
Daily Totals	**179**	**45**	**195**	**2651**

STEVE: Phase IV Meal Plan for Workout Days				
Contents	**Protein** (grams)	**Carbs** (grams)	**Fats** (grams)	**Calories**
First Solid Meal P+F Gourmet omelet of 6 whole eggs, ½ tbsp coconut oil, spinach, mixed veggies, 3 turkey sausages, and low-carb hot sauce	95	0	48	821
Para-Workout Beverage P+C Workout Beverage—3 scoops BioTrust Low-Carb mixed with 12 oz fat-free milk. Consume ⅔ of this drink during the second half of your workout. Finish immediately upon completion.	50	30	5	365
Dinner Meal P+C+F 1 large filet mignon, 2 slices peameal bacon, tossed tomato, cabbage, cucumber, radish, ½ cup sauerkraut, 3 medium baked potatoes with salt and butter	95	130	50	1350
Daily Totals	**240**	**160**	**103**	**2536**

STEVE: Phase IV Meal Plan for Non-Workout Days				
Contents	**Protein** (grams)	**Carbs** (grams)	**Fats** (grams)	**Calories**
First Solid Meal P+F 4 medium-large chicken thighs, seaweed salad with lemon and herbs, extra veggies as desired	53	0	38	554
Midday Meal P+C+F Medium-large steak of kangaroo or boar, onions fried in organic butter, kale and baby greens salad with tomato and 1 tbsp macadamia nut oil	53	0	38	554
Dinner Meal P+C+F Medium-large turkey breast, 1 serving organic pesto, 1 cup jasmine rice fried in organic butter with chopped broccoli and choice of spices.	54	40	39	727
Daily Totals	**160**	**40**	**115**	**1835**

PHASE IV WORKOUTS

	Monday	Tuesday	Wednesday	Thursday	Friday	Saturday	Sunday
			Complete Training Schedule				
Week 1	Workout 1	OFF	Workout 2	OFF	Workout 3	OFF	OFF
Week 2	Workout 4	OFF	Workout 1	OFF	Workout 2	OFF	OFF
Week 3	Workout 3	OFF	Workout 4	OFF	Workout 2	OFF	OFF
Week 4	Workout 1	OFF	Workout 4	OFF	Workout 3	OFF	OFF

PHASE IV, WORKOUT 1

A Rack Pulls from the Knee
20 reps

This is a 20-rep set done at a steady tempo with challenging weight. After this set, rest 2–3 minutes and proceed to workout set B.

B1 Low-Incline Dumbbell Bench Press
12 reps

B2 Seated Row
10 reps

B3 Plank
Hold for 60 seconds

The first two exercises are performed lactic-acid style at a tempo of 4-0-1 for 10–12 reps each, a total of 3 times. Select a weight appropriate for each exercise (often, different weights each circuit). Tempo does not factor in for the plank. Simply hold for 60 seconds.

Perform exercises B1–B3 sequentially, resting 10–30 seconds between exercises. After B3, rest 90 seconds and repeat. After your last circuit, rest 2 minutes and proceed to workout set C.

C1 **Lateral Raise**
12 reps

C2 **Dumbbell Romanian Deadlift**
8 reps

◗ Grab a pair of dumbbells with an overhand grip, and hold them at arm's length in front of your thighs. Stand with your feet hip-width apart and your knees slightly bent.

◗ Without changing the bend in your knees, bend at your hips and lower your torso until it's almost parallel to the floor.

◗ Pause, then raise your torso back to the starting position.

These two exercises are performed at a tempo of 4-0-1 for 8–12 reps each, a total of 4 times. Select a weight appropriate for each exercise (often, different weights each circuit). Perform exercises C1–C2 sequentially, resting 10 seconds between exercises. After C3, rest 90 seconds and repeat. After your last set, rest 2 minutes and proceed to workout set D.

D **Rack Pulls from the Knee**
25 reps

This is *not* a lactic acid–based exercise. This is a 25-rep set done with only your body weight.

PHASE IV, WORKOUT 2

A1 **Dumbbell Alpha Press**
8 reps

A2 **Alpha Deadlift**
6 reps

A3 **Barbell Bent-Over Row**
8 reps

A4 **Hanging Knee Raise**
10 reps

Perform A1–A4 in a circuit fashion, resting no more than 30 seconds between exercises. Perform 5 circuits, resting 3 minutes between each.

B **Two-Arm Kettlebell Swing**
30–45 seconds

Perform 3 sets of 30–45 seconds of Kettlebell Swings, resting 2 minutes between each. After your last set, rest 2 minutes and proceed to the next circuit.

C1 **Push-Up**
12–15 reps

C2 **Jump Squat**
10 reps

C3 **Plank**
30 seconds

Perform C1–C3 in a circuit fashion, resting no more than 15 seconds between exercises. Perform 2 circuits, resting 15 seconds between exercises and 30 seconds between sets.

PHASE IV, WORKOUT 3

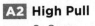 **Trap Bar Deadlift**
6–8 reps

A2 **High Pull**
6–8 reps

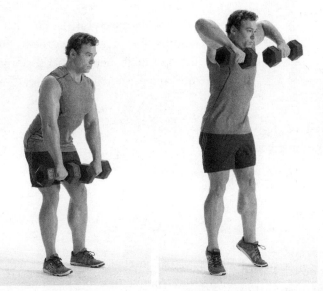

♦ Grab a pair of dumbbells with an overhand grip and hold them just above knee height.

♦ Explosively pull the dumbbells upward, rise onto your toes, and bend your elbows as you bring the weights up to shoulder height. Return to the starting position.

♦ Weight selection: pick a weight you could lift 8–12 times.

Alternate A1 and A2 for 5 minutes. The goal is to get as many reps as possible. After this circuit, rest 3–5 minutes. Then increase weights by 5 to 10 percent and repeat the circuit for another 5 minutes. After the second time through, rest another 3–5 minutes and proceed to workout set B.

B1 **Reverse Lunge**
6–8 reps

B2 **Face Pull**
6–8 reps

B3 **Standing Dumbbell Overhead Press**
6–8 reps

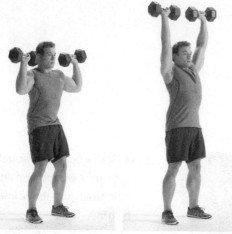

▶ Weight selection: pick a weight you could lift 12–15 times.

Cycle through B1, B2, and B3 for 6 minutes. The goal is to get as many reps as possible. After this circuit, rest 3–5 minutes. Then increase weights by 3 to 5 percent and repeat the circuit for another 6 minutes. After the second time through, rest another 3–5 minutes and proceed to workout set C.

C1 **Rear Delt Fly**
6–8 reps

C2 **Reverse Curl**
6–8 reps

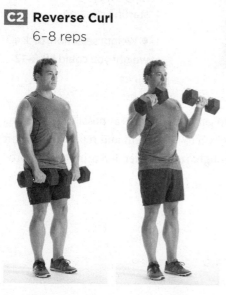

▶ Grab a pair of dumbbells with an overhand, shoulder-width grip so that your palms are angled slightly inward.

▶ The dumbbells should hang at arm's length in front of your waist. Without moving your upper arms, bend your elbows and curl the dumbbells as close to your shoulders as you can.

▶ Pause, then lower the weight back to the starting position.

▶ Weight selection: pick a weight you could lift 8–12 times.

Alternate C1 and C2 for 4 minutes. The goal is to get as many reps as possible. After this circuit, rest 2 minutes. Then repeat the circuit for another 5 minutes with the same weight.

PHASE IV, WORKOUT 4

A1 **Barbell Front Squat**
5 reps

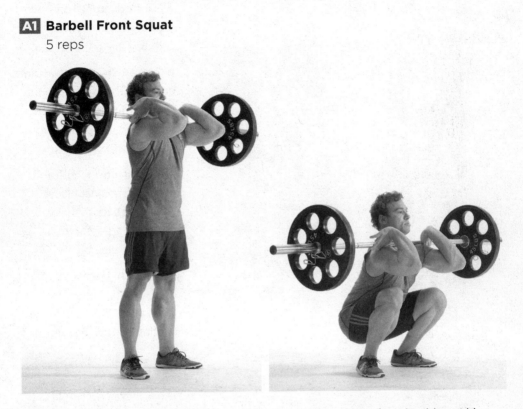

◈ Hold a barbell across your upper chest with a clean grip and your feet shoulder-width apart.

◈ Keeping your lower back arched, lower your body as deep as you can by pushing your hips back and bending your knees.

◈ Pause, then reverse the movement back to the starting position.

A2 Weighted Chin-Up
5 reps

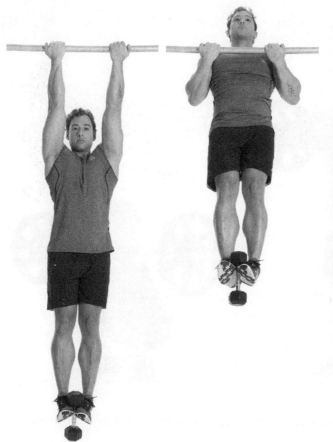

◉ Place a dumbbell on the floor underneath a chin-up bar.

◉ Grab a chin-up bar with an underhand grip that's about shoulder-width apart, and then "hold" the dumbbell in your feet.

◉ Hang at arm's length and pull your shoulder blades down and back so that your shoulders are as far from your ears as possible.

◉ Hold at the top position for a second, then slowly lower your body back to the starting position and repeat.

Alternate A1 and A2 for a total of 5 sets each. There is no need to time your rest periods, but try to get back to work when you feel you're fully recovered. For most people, that's 2 minutes between sets.

Pick a weight that you can complete 5 reps with on the first set. The weight should be challenging, and, in fact, you shouldn't be able to complete 5 reps on all 5 sets. For instance, you might complete 5 reps on the first two sets, and then 3 reps, 2 reps, and 1 rep. If you complete fewer than 14 total reps on an exercise, lower the weight; otherwise stay at the same weight as you perform more total reps with each passing week. If you can perform 25 or more total reps, then increase the weight you're using.

After your last set, proceed to workout set B.

B1 Barbell Bench Press
5 reps

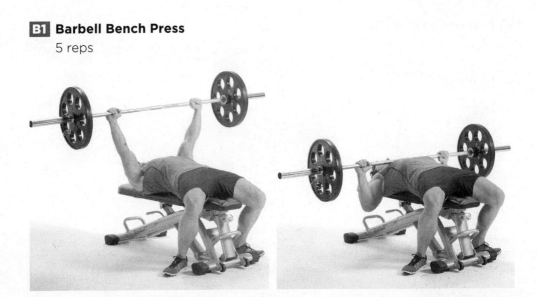

◗ Lie on your back on a bench. Grasp a barbell with an overhand grip that's just wider than shoulder-width and hold it above your sternum with your arms completely straight.

◗ Lower the bar straight down in a controlled fashion. Make sure you keep your elbows tucked in close to your body so your upper arms form a 45-degree angle to your body in the down position.

◗ Pause, and then press the bar in a straight line back up to the starting position.

B2 Alpha Deadlift
5 reps

Alternate B1 and B2 for a total of 5 sets each. There is no need to time your rest periods, but try to get back to work when you feel you're fully recovered. For most people, that's 2 minutes.

Pick a weight that you can complete 5 reps with on the first set. The weight should be challenging, and, in fact, you shouldn't be able to complete 5 reps on all 5 sets. For instance, you might complete 5 reps on the first two sets, and then 3 reps, 2 reps, and 1 rep. If you complete fewer than 14 total reps on an exercise, lower the weight; otherwise stay at the same weight as you perform more total reps with each passing week. If you can perform 25 or more total reps, then increase the weight you're using.

I, Alpha

TAKING THE FIRST STEP AS A NEW MAN AND MAKING IT LAST

"A man is a success if he gets up in the morning and goes to bed at night and in between does what he wants to do."
—BOB DYLAN

"Follow your bliss."
—JOSEPH CAMPBELL

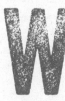hen you began this journey, you were a permanent inhabitant of the Ordinary World and—at best—a visitor and outsider to the Special World.

Despite having a place that felt familiar, you never really had a place to call your own. That's because you were searching, hoping, or wanting a life that was better. A life that was incredible. A life that was Alpha.

And now, after having the courage to follow our steps, this became your journey. What started as a story about our lessons has become a book about you and the influence you'll have on your world and others. This is about *your* ability to rise up and become stronger. And your decision to accept that a good life is great, but an unreal life is the true quest of the Alpha.

Your individual rise will spark a charge that can put an end to the current state of the ordinary man. Your ability to become Alpha—to be confident, assertive, and driven to help others is what will make you a better man, and this world a better place.

Whether you realized it or not, this has been your goal from the beginning. When you picked up this book, it was an acknowledgment of a desire to reach Apotheosis and become the best version of yourself. Now that you're here, you should take pride in what you've accomplished.

Reaching a moment of Apotheosis isn't a given; it's something that requires work and struggles. In order to reach Apotheosis, the hero must go through the Ordeal. This is the final step on the Road of Trials, and it's your ultimate challenge. It's the big boss at the end of the video game or the final battle in any movie.

For you, that battle is both internal and external. During the course of the next sixteen weeks, you'll be engaging in battle every day—with both your body and your mind. You'll have to calm your concerns, ignore what you "know" as reason, and abstain from your old behaviors. You'll have to challenge your body and do workouts that might be harder than anything you've done in your entire life. You'll have to integrate a new diet approach that, while extremely beneficial and enjoyable in time, can have a difficult adjustment period.

These are challenges meant to shape and change you—tools that you can use to metaphorically kill the old version of yourself so the Alpha version can arise.

By accepting and embracing fear and not backing down, you'll reach Apotheosis. You'll experience a moment when you realize that you can change anything in your life. If you can change your body, why not your job? If you can abstain from bad food decisions, why can't you avoid bad decisions with women? If you can consistently make your way to the gym, why can't you consistently find happiness in your life?

We don't mean to imply a direct correlation between visiting the gym and happiness, but the dedication needed to seek self-improvement is no different than the effort needed to achieve happiness. And that's the parallel you need to draw with the decisions you've made and the person you will now become. Any success you create for yourself should build confidence to create other success. And because nothing is more challenging or inherently tied to your sense of being than your own body, mastery over your appearance is the catalyst for confidence, success, and happiness in any and all areas of your life.

THE ALPHA REVOLUTION

This is what happens when you've joined us at one of the final stages of the Hero's Journey: the Ultimate Boon.

During this phase the hero either receives or gives a gift to the world at the conclusion of the final battle. Sometimes it's tangible like a chest of gold or a magic sword; other times it's intangible like bringing peace to the world or reestablishing balance to the Force.

To an Alpha, the Ultimate Boon is knowledge. It's both tangible and intangible. The tangible aspect is your new body. Your hormones will be optimized. Your mind and body will function better than ever. And you'll be healthier from the inside out. But you already know that. What you now must realize is that not only do you know how to build and maintain your body, but you also know how to help others.

As your body changes, you'll start to be asked—constantly—about what you're doing and how you're making these radical shifts. Now you are *the* inspiration to others. Your transition to the Alpha will empower your friends, family, and peers to begin their own journey and *believe* they can have success. Remember, psychological hurdles are oftentimes the biggest barriers, but your presence as the Alpha can help others overcome that significant obstacle.

One of our success stories, Claudio, lost more than sixty pounds of fat, gained twelve pounds of muscle, and added thirty to forty pounds to every single one of his lifts. For Claudio, those were the tangible benefits. However, the intangible rewards began to surface too. We keep in touch with all our clients, and to date, Claudio has inspired four of his friends to get in shape. Not by speaking of his program or convincing them, but just by living the Alpha lifestyle. That presence made his friends want to begin their own journey. Two of those friends signed up to be coached by us, and a third has lost 100 pounds on his own.

Claudio's transformation—the death of his old body and the rise of a new one from its ashes—has inspired everyone around him to live a better life. That is the greatest gift you can give to others—and one of the distinguishing factors that separates Alphas from a-holes; you can help others accomplish what you achieve during this program.

I'M ALPHA, SO WHAT'S NEXT?

The next-to-last phase is the Master of Two Worlds. In mythology, this is a character that can live in the physical and spiritual worlds after reaching Apotheosis. For you, it means actively balancing the demands of the Ordinary World that you have left and the Alpha World you have entered. At the conclusion of the program, many of our clients are unsure what to do. The most natural question is, should I continue on the program?

If you choose to continue on this program, that's fine. But we recognize that many people feel like they are ready for something else. And yet the fear exists that, if you are no longer following our plan, you will be unable to stay on track.

Don't fear that. Remember, you're a new man now. You don't need us.* You just need to remember the lessons you learned and remind yourself of the person you are.

You are *Alpha*. You've gone through all the stages. You've confronted all the challenges that have held back men stuck in the Ordinary World. The hard work is done. You have to see your track record of success, your willingness to venture into the unknown, and your ability to lead others down the same path.

You no longer need us because now you are us. You are the Alpha.

---

* While you don't need us, we definitely want you to become a member of our community. Head to engineering thealpha.com to get everything from the latest tips and strategies to extra workouts, completely free.

You know the Seven Traits of the Alpha. You can balance cockiness and confidence, and you understand the difference between vanity and conceit. Most importantly, you are in control.

And because you are in control, you will be able to enter the final stage of the journey—Freedom to Live—with confidence. This is sometimes known as living in the moment, as you'll possess a new mind-set in which you're neither anxious about the future nor regretting your past.

Experiencing Freedom to Live means that you are free from the ties that previously prevented you from being happy and living the life you want. The Alpha realizes that fortune favors the bold and that any great achievement comes with the risk of failure. But after going through this process, you now understand that failure isn't a bad thing; it's a necessary step on the path to success. You know this because you are the Alpha. You have gone through the trials and overcome the hurdles on your path, and you now understand that this is the ultimate truth.

More than anything, you will feel in control of your body and more in control of your life and what you can accomplish. You won't have those nagging questions that have burned inside us all: Is there something more? Can my life be better? Those uncertainties arrive when you are a visitor in a land that doesn't feel like your own. That was then; this is now. Now, you have the knowledge and wherewithal to create the life you want and face anything—the good and the bad—with an unshakable swagger.

Armed with that knowledge, fortified with that swagger, you'll become who and what you were always meant to be. If we may be so bold as to paraphrase Tyler Durden once more, you are now ready to look how you want to look and fuck how you want to fuck; you're smarter, more capable and free in ways that you were not. That last part is the most important: you're free to do anything.

Think big. Think bold. Kick some ass and do what you've always wanted. You have the mind and the body built to take on the world with the type of confidence needed to succeed. Your reality is no longer clouded with questions but rather is open and free. A canvas of unprecedented and limitless opportunity awaits you . . . *the hero*. The present and your future have never looked better.

Welcome home, Alpha.

Acknowledgments

To the HarperOne Team: You are first class. Mark Tauber, thank you for your faith in us. To Claudia Boutote, Laina Adler, Michele Wetherbee, Terri Leonard, Lisa Zuniga, Terry McGrath, Dwight Been, Suzanne Wickham, and Elsa Dixon, your contributions and hard work made this come to life. And to Nancy Hancock, our incredibly talented editor: you made this book so much better and found a way to keep our profanity at a professional level.
—Roman and Born

The thanks and gratitude for writing this book extend in so many directions that it's hard to quantify my extreme appreciation to everyone who has made a difference. I'll start with my co-author and friend, John Romaniello. No other man was more suited to help me create a guide that would redefine the meaning of Alpha, and open the door for so many men to improve their lives.

I must extend my humble appreciation to Arnold Schwarzenegger for his continued support and belief in me. Scott Hoffman, you are the best book agent an author could ask for.

The following have been incredible mentors and guides in fitness, nutrition, and personal wellness: Jason Ferruggia, Jim Smith, Martin Rooney, Alwyn Cosgrove, Craig Ballantyne, Eric Cressey, Bill Hartman, Mike Robertson, Alan Aragon, John Berardi, Bret Contreras, Nick Tumminello, David Jack, Robert Dos Remedios, Dan Trink, Rob Sulaver, and Clifton Harski.

And those who made me a better writer, editor, and businessman: Lewis Howes, Mike Zimmerman, Jason Feifer, Sean Hyson, Jeff O'Connell, Derek Flanzraich, and Dan Brian. Dave Forsberg, Joseph O'Neill, Quinn Sypniewski, and Daniel Ketchel: You are great friends who deserve more than one line. Ted Spiker, you're the ultimate mentor and friend. Neema Yazdani: This all started ten years ago. I couldn't have unleashed my inner Alpha without you.

Josh, Aaron, and Jordan: I wish everyone could have brothers as awesome as you. You are the best source of testosterone, humility, and confidence I know of. My parents: Ira and Sandra. I dedicated this book to you, but nothing will ever be enough to thank you for all your love and support.

And finally, Rachie. Every day has been an unreal life since I met you. Thank you for being my world and my #1. You are beyond amazing. I love you.
—AB

I must start with my mother; for her hard work and sacrifice in raising two children, including a son who caused all the pain that I did. Thank you, Mom, for teaching me goodness and honor, but also doggedness and work ethic, and doing your best to raise me to believe I could do anything. Thank you also for trying to teach me some humility; I'm sorry that it didn't take.

To my sister Jessica, the only person who can ever really understand my childhood. Thank you for being a touchstone to my past, and not posting anything overly embarrassing on the Internet.

To my Miyagi, Alvin Batista: you taught me so much of what is in this book. From you, I learned about training and women and being a good man—and sometimes, how to be not so good.

I must thank all of my friends who saw me barely survive boyhood to grasp at manhood. Adam, John, Chis, Mike, Tom, Josh, Rob, Ross, Evan, and the Brothers Trott. Thank you for having my back, and seeing through my mistakes.

To Joel Marion, Eric Cressey, Eric Chessen, and all the RUGGED crew. Who knew we'd eventually figure this out? To Joel especially, I owe my thanks and much of my success. Thank you for seeing so much in me. To Craig Ballantyne, Vince and Flavia Del Monte, Jeff Siegal and Isabel De Los Rios, Alex Maroko, Jason Ferruggia, Adam Steer, Matt McGorry, Ryan Murdock, Sirena Bernal, Lewis Howes, and everyone in the Internet Marketing crowd; whatever success I've had, I owe to all of you. Thank you so much for your friendship.

To my clients past and present: A sincere *thank you* to everyone who didn't run away when I said, "today we're going to try an experiment." Thanks to anyone who has read a blog or clicked a link or bought a product. You made this dream real. The RFS team: starting with David Sinick, who made sure I hit my deadlines; and Josh and Rob, for running my business while I was bleeding on pages.

To early mentors: TC Luoma, the first editor to give me my first shot; and Dr. John Berardi, who gave far too generously of his wisdom and time. I'll never be able to express my gratitude. And more recent mentors: Tim Ferriss, Gary Vaynerchuk, Tucker Max, Neil Strauss, and Ryan Holiday. Your work is a constant inspiration. And I must thank Arnold Schwarzenegger, for all you have done for the industry, for me, and for this book.

I must thank Adam Bornstein, my friend and co-author; I could not ask for a more stalwart friend to have at my back. Working with you has made me a better writer and a better man.

Finally, we come to the end. Here, I must thank my muse, Neghar Fonooni. My *anam cara,* my Scheherazade, my best friend: no paltry words of mine can ever express the *grace* of knowing you. From my lips you have drawn so many things that I cannot thank you for them all. But for your constant support, and gentle reminders that *luminous beings are we,* I do thank you, and forever will.

Thank you all.

Snuggles,

John Romaniello

Index

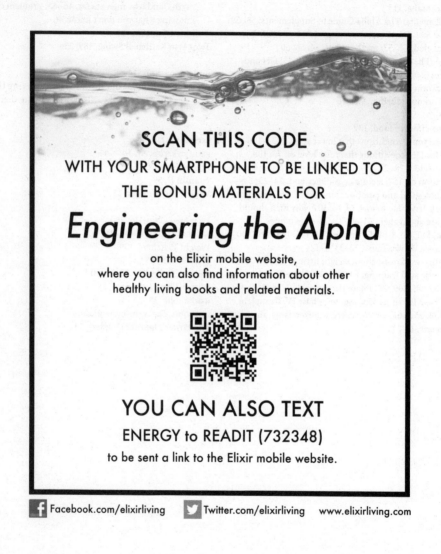